The Endurance Paradox

The Endurance Paradox

Bone Health for the Endurance Athlete

Thomas J. Whipple

Robert B. Eckhardt

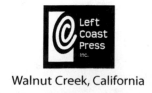

Left Coast Press
Inc.

Walnut Creek, California

LEFT COAST PRESS, INC.
1630 North Main Street, #400
Walnut Creek, CA 94596
http://www.LCoastPress.com

ISBN 978-1-59874-617-4 hardback
ISBN 978-1-61132-785-4 paperback
ISBN 978-1-59874-618-1 institutional eBook
ISBN 978-1-61132-490-4 consumer eBook

Library of Congress Cataloging-in-Publication Data:

Whipple, Thomas J.
   The endurance paradox : bone health for the endurance athlete / Thomas
J. Whipple and Robert B. Eckhardt.
      p. ; cm.
   Includes bibliographical references and index.
   ISBN 978-1-59874-617-4 (hardback : alk. paper)—ISBN 978-1-61132-785-4
(paperback : alk. paper)—ISBN 978-1-59874-618-1 (institutional eBook)
—ISBN 978-1-61132-490-4 (consumer eBook)

1. Athletes--Nutrition. 2. Physical fitness—Nutritional aspects.
3. Stress fractures (Orthopedics) 4. Bioenergetics. I. Eckhardt, Robert B.
II. Title. [DNLM: 1. Physical Endurance. 2. Bone and Bones. 3. Fractures,
Stress—rehabilitation. 4. Nutritional Physiological Phenomena—physiology.
QT 255]
   TX361.A8W45 2011
   613.2'024796–dc22

2010052552

Printed in the United States of America

∞™ The paper used in this publication meets the minimum requirements
of American National Standard for Information Sciences—Permanence of
Paper for Printed Library Materials, ANSI/NISO Z39.48–1992.

Cover design by Piper Wallis

CONTENTS

FOREWORD

It is widely accepted that endurance exercise is beneficial to our health and well-being. However, it has also become fairly well known that extreme exercise can have negative effects on nutrition, hormonal balance, and ultimately bone health, and that these effects may not be reversible. As a former athlete and coach, and now as a physician, understanding the science behind how exercise can affect health—and how health can affect exercise performance—has always been one of the most interesting and important aspects of sports medicine and one that has always engaged me. Understanding that "exercise is medicine" and seeing how different medical conditions can play a role in exercise performance and health is what led me to pursue a career in primary care sports medicine and to my work as a team physician.

How can exercise promote health, well-being, and strong bones, but in the extreme lead to fatigue, poor performance, stress fractures, and premature osteopenia? This book provides the answers and shows how athletes can implement changes to optimize bone health, and ultimately overall health and performance.

The Endurance Paradox is a tremendously useful resource for athletes, coaches, and strength and conditioning coaches, as well as for the wide variety of people who care for athletes—parents, athletic trainers, physical therapists, physicians, and other health care providers. Authors Thomas Whipple and Robert Eckhardt use a scientific approach to each topic and incorporate the most recent research on endurance athletes. They present this information in a format that is easy to understand and apply; each chapter is a guide that athletes can use to improve their bone health as well as their overall health and performance.

As a sports medicine physician, I welcome this resource for the sports medicine community. It speaks directly to athletes and those

7

around them in a manner that is refreshing and honest. I congratulate the authors and editors for a job well done.

Margot Putukian, MD, FACSM

Director of Athletic Medicine, Head Team Physician, Princeton University

Associate Clinical Professor, Robert Wood Johnson, UMDNJ

Past President, American Medical Society for Sports Medicine

FOREWORD

This book is useful as a fundamental training guide for endurance athletes of all levels. The information it offers is increasingly urgent because, as the authors pointed out, athletes are experiencing skeletal ageing and premature bone loss at accelerating rates. This book can help athletes reverse that trend and decrease their risk.

Richard Feynman has said, "A paradox is not a conflict with reality. It is a conflict between reality and your feelings of what reality should be like." This perspective applies to the field of endurance, in which a paradigm of cardiovascular development has become so dominant that it is leading to the deterioration of health and performance. What athletes were trying to achieve by emphasizing their endurance performance came at the cost of athleticism elsewhere.

At the beginning of the running boom of the 1970s, neither athletes nor coaches were paying enough attention to strength development for runners. To get better at running, they thought, you just have to run more. Instead of providing for the overall development of the human organism, they focused on the cardiovascular and respiratory systems as the keys to enhanced performance. High volumes of training, they believed, would improve these systems and result in faster marathon performances. However, the results were not faster times, but generations of broken runners. The combination of high mileage along with poor technique and the absence of strength training was a formula for disaster.

By the end of the 1970s, a fractional group of enlightened coaches began to rethink strength training and started recommending weight programs for their runners. While mainstream runners are still behind this trend, the efforts of leading scientists and coaches are being acknowledged and the value of strength conditioning for achieving endurance running results has been undeniably proven. The authors of this book are among those scientists who clearly understand the value of strength training for endurance athletes. Their literature review does not leave any doubt about the importance of strength training and provides you with noteworthy guidance in this direction.

But the book covers much more. The curious reader will find other enlightening information and will learn how quality training programs should be supplemented with technique, diet, and other program mainstays. The book leads readers to a profound understanding of it and makes recommendations for solving them. It covers a very wide spectrum of aspects of training and wellbeing, from strength training and nutrition to metabolism and rehabilitation. I think it is an invaluable source of information for everyone interested in endurance performance.

Nicholas Romanov, PhD
Founder of the Pose Method

FOREWORD

Life is a challenge of compromises. One thing more here usually means something less there. If that isn't sobering enough, consider a paradox: you might be investing "everything" in order to achieve a desired result, only to find out later that this effort actually reduced rather than increased your chances of reaching your goal.

Endurance athletes are painfully aware of the problematic payoff game: we are nurtured on the dual dogmas of innate talent on the one hand, and the idea that our allotted payoff will be pretty much in direct proportion to our physical effort on the other. These dogmas keep us going sometimes until we drop—literally—or end up with poorer performance, and injury, and maybe in the long-term with accentuated frailty of the bones. Meanwhile, we see someone who appears to put half as much heart into the enterprise achieve twice the glory.

All of our actions and goals demand the application of method, not just brute force. But to follow through with sustained vigor also requires the confidence that we are using the best possible methods. As runners we struggle to find our way, especially beyond the age when we automatically relied on authority figures for guidance. We tend to rely mostly on hearsay and examples of what has worked or not worked for others and for ourselves. We all are different and we continually change with age and experiences. Our goals change as well. Paradoxically, a positive result now may produce a negative one at some later time, and vice versa.

We are confronted with a welter of variables, making the achievement of specific results more art than science, and I suspect it will continue to be an art at the personal level. However, as much as the art of running makes it interesting and challenging, the more science we can apply to our thinking and planning, the more variables are revealed that we had not even thought of and the more choices we have. The science now available from countless controlled studies provides an understanding of the underlying physiological mechanisms that, in turn, provide a framework for generating desired results and reducing or eliminating undesired consequences.

The Endurance Paradox by Thomas Whipple and Robert Eckhardt draws on current research to give answers to age-old problems that all runners face. As a former insect physiologist and still-practicing runner I learned much and appreciated it greatly.

Bernd Heinrich, PhD

Professor Emeritus
Department of Biology,
University of Vermont

United States Ultramarathon
Record Holder

ACKNOWLEDGMENTS

Tom:
My deepest thanks and appreciation go to the following people who contributed, directly or indirectly, to the development of this book: My parents, especially my Mom, whose presence is missed daily; my past clinical and academic mentors Dan Greenwood, Robert Hensel, Douglas Jackson, John Eckhold, Gordon Cummings, Jerry Lee, and Mark Albert, thank you for your guidance and willingness to share of yourselves during my most impressionable professional years; my past colleagues in Atlanta, Peter Spiegel and Robert Medcalf, for whom I credit with providing me the steepest clinical learning curve in my 20 plus years of practice; my past and present colleagues at Penn State Sports Medicine, especially Dean Plafcan, John Miller, Craig Denegar, Susan Fix, Chris Hurd, Jennifer Reed, Brian Schultz, Sally Bondurant, and Tonya Confer, for the lessons in balance that you all seem to have created between an absolute dedication to the clinic and the selflessness of your personal and family pursuits; my Penn State University associates, Nancy Williams, Mary Jane De Souza, John Challis, and Neil Sharkey, thank you for your generosity of time and resources with which you so freely share; to Lawrence Demers for providing me with the opportunity to learn from true leader in skeletal biochemistry and to experience the operations of a world class clinical laboratory at the Hershey Medical Center; to Dr. Brian Le for both your laboratory mentorship and assistance in manuscript preparation; to the Physicians that have entrusted me with the care of their patients; especially Doug Aukerman, Phil Bosha, John Deitch, Paul Sherbondy, and Bobbi Millard; to Wayne Sebastianelli and Lori Benner for allowing me the time and support necessary to expand my professional pursuits; to the many coaches that have shared their expertise and insightful perspectives, especially Nicholas Romanov

and Harry Groves; to the elite athletes that have so willingly provided their empirical experiences, especially Dr. Francesca Conte, and Xeno Mueller; to the patients that have provided both inspiration and my most important source of education; to my friends Steve Cox, Ben Tartell, and Paul Cutler who have enriched my life by sharing their experiences and unique types of endurance; to my co-author Bob Eckhardt, a sincere thanks for such a welcoming agreement for collaboration as well as for your contagious sense of optimism; and lastly to my wife, Jody for her steadfast confidence and never ending support that has enabled our relationship to grow stronger, our children Jacob and Abbey to feel the love of two parents when I have been absent, and the idea for this book to become a reality.

Bob:
My intellectual obligations to others might comprise a volume of modest length all in itself, and of necessity would include a very great many teachers, mentors, colleagues, students, friends, and family members. Only the few most salient of these contributors can be noted here. First must be Tom Whipple, who drew me into a publishing endeavor that very much is his own, but which I feel privileged to have had a chance in helping shape to some modest extent. The more conventional list of those to whom I am indebted would have to include Joseph E. Slater, Donald S. Douglas, and Charlotte J. Avers, all in my undergraduate years. Joseph Slater was my instructor in a first year honors section of English Composition at Rutgers. His once per week very late afternoon seminar meetings of several hours with 10 or so students, each time discussing the weekly essays required in his course, probably came about as close as one might in a public university to the extremely effective Oxbridge tutorial system. That the year's work centered on the writings of George Orwell, particularly his essays, probably was more than just the happy accident it seemed at the time. In my estimation Orwell is the greatest essayist in the English language, and in later years I gradually have come to realize that Slater knew that he was teaching a group that included not only English majors but one or two of us who had strayed in from the sciences, and that even we might be persuaded that attention to literary style could have value anywhere. It was from Donald Douglas that I acquired my groundwork in physiology and, more unusually, an appreciation for the great value of concise writing in science. At Rutgers' College of Agriculture in his time, physiology was taught at least as much in the laboratory as in lectures. Don conducted our long afternoon labs with extensive preparation and great attention throughout. What is more, week after week he carefully

read our lab reports (commonly 20 or so pages) and commented extensively on them. Formulation of hypotheses and their testing was central; clarity and economy of expression were the expected norms. Charlotte Avers was Professor and Chair of Biology at Douglass College. Until writing these acknowledgments I had not realized that the year (1964) in which I was a finishing senior at Rutgers University and took her graduate course in Physiological Genetics was her first there; everything about the course, and the discipline, seemed just to be reflexively natural to her. Of all my teachers during undergraduate school she was simultaneously the most sternly demanding yet positively stimulating; uncompromising high standards work to create that combination. Her untimely death from cancer, like that of Rosalind Franklin before her, took a great scientist far too early from the world. At Michigan, Frank B. Livingstone, Ernst Goldschmidt, and Alan G. Fix in Anthropology, Charles Radding in Human Genetics, and Norman E. Nelson in English were the primary collegial influences on me in graduate school, and their contributions were far too disparate to summarize economically. Similarly, Gerald E. Mc Clearn, Karl M. Newell, Robert L. Sainburg, and Robert K. Selander continue to be major intellectual influences on me at Penn State. Especially great thanks of another sort are due to Maciej Henneberg and John Schofield, co-authors of another book, *The Hobbit Trap*, on which the three of us have been working through much of this year, and thanks largely to their efforts now just has gone to press; their patience with my attention and writing divided between the two books is a gift that will not be forgotten. Those many other valued colleagues who do not see their names on the page here nonetheless will know where they stand on a special roster in my mind. Anyone trained in genetics must be cognizant of biological and cultural contributions, both known and unknown, made by family members including not only parents but also their parents and so on back through millennia. In what species other than ours could a special, direct, and independent obligation be owed to the parent of a mate, as is mine to my wife's father, Joseph Davis? Then, too, what goes around, comes around: among those living, by now I have learned and benefited more from my sons, David and Jonathan, than I believe ever they have from me. To Carey, my wife, most valued confidante and daily beloved companion of more than 46 years, I ask only that there be another such fleeting period ahead for both of us.

INTRODUCTION

Endurance exercise has the potential to improve the quality and quantity of life for people of all ages. However, there is a paradox, since many athletes experience accelerated rates of skeletal ageing and premature bone loss. This unfortunate and often preventable trend is being recognized more frequently in adolescents and adults who participate in sports such as swimming, cycling, running, rowing, and other ultra endurance activities including hiking and adventure racing. The purpose of *The Endurance Paradox* is to provide athletes and those who care for them with a comprehensive resource for preventing and managing exercise-related bone loss as well as maximizing long-term skeletal health and performance.

In our clinical practice, we are treating exercise-induced stress fractures and osteoporosis at an alarming rate. Although many athletes understand how endurance training influences their race performances and cardio-respiratory systems, there appears to be a shortage of information regarding the consequences of these actions on the skeleton. Bone is a dynamic structure that is capable of undergoing *acute* and *chronic* adaptations in response to the actions of two specialized bone cell types. The cells that liberate *calcium* from storage and dissolve (resorb) old or damaged bone are known as *osteoclasts* while those that form new bone are *osteoblasts*. The actions of these cells are linked, or "coupled," but the net result of their respective actions is a product of influences from multiple factors, many of which are amenable to specific training and lifestyle strategies. The primary governors of bone cell activity include mechanical loads, induced by exercising muscles or ground reaction forces, as well as various nutritional and hormonal states. Other exercise-related stresses that are known to influence bone cell activity include alterations in acid-base balance, dehydration, and emotional distress. Understanding how these variables can affect the skeleton is necessary to minimize the risk of bone loss and maximize general health and performance.

The skeleton undergoes net bone loss when the rate or degree of bone *resorption* exceeds that of formation, while gains in bone strength and mass occur when the reverse is true. During normal development, bone gain typically is positive through early adulthood, at which time *peak bone mass* is achieved. Throughout midlife bone loss and gain tend to be steady: only slight reductions in mass are considered normal. During the late adulthood years, bone loss accelerates, especially in females, as the overall rate of resorption increases relative to formation.

Why does the skeleton remodel? Like all other tissues, bone attempts to adapt to its environment in a manner that is consistent with providing an individual the greatest chance of survival. Functional short-term reactions to physical or emotional stress, including the loss of calcium from bone, may become pathologic if sustained or repeated too frequently. The rate at which bone can be lost or damaged can change in minutes or hours and often is dependent upon such factors as local muscle fatigue, exercise intensity, or calcium and vitamin D availability. In contrast, the time required for a cycle of *bone remodeling* and formation to occur is on the order of three months. Because of this temporal discrepancy between the rates at which resorption and formation processes proceed, the opportunity for bone loss and resultant risk of fracture is substantial.

Just as every athlete is unique, the particular combinations of factors that accelerate each individual's bone loss also may be unique; however, typically there are several common findings. The classic example that routinely is cited in female athletes is a reduction in the hormone *estrogen*. Other common factors that may undermine skeletal health in both male and female athletes include inadequate dietary energy, carbohydrate and sodium loading, insufficient dietary protein, or the intensity and duration of exercise. Further considerations we will discuss include losses of muscular strength and *power*, elevated levels of systemic inflammation, and excessive *free radical* formation.

To provide readers with a comprehensive resource, we have included extensive scientific references as well as empirical evidence and case studies from a variety of sports. *The Endurance Paradox* is not so much a how-to manual as it is a reference that we hope will serve to enlighten readers on how certain aspects of endurance training, competition, and lifestyle may be considered in the context of long-term musculoskeletal health. We hope that you will find the information both relevant and practical, and look forward to the opportunity of expanding this work based upon your shared experiences. We invite you to post your comments with us at enduranceorthopaedics.com.

CHAPTER ONE

Strength Training

The Muscle-Bone Connection

It may seem paradoxical that the cardiovascular and pulmonary systems respond favorably to progressively larger exercise volumes while your muscles and bones actually may become weaker. Even though you may experience improved fatigue resistance and therefore feel "stronger" as you add meters or miles to your weekly training log, the forces acting on bones remain relatively consistent and don't increase substantially in magnitude. From a mechanical perspective, the forces acting on the skeleton during endurance exercise are relatively small when compared to those generated during other types of sports.

The largest forces encountered by our bones are those associated with vigorous muscle contractions and with the ground reaction forces associated with landing. Intriguingly, studies of weight lifters and gymnasts reveal that these groups have significantly higher levels of muscle strength and therefore *bone mass* than do endurance athletes. Consider the forces on the skeleton that are associated with barbell squatting while bearing 800 pounds, or dismounting from the uneven bars! In comparison to strength and power athletes, endurance specialists score well below average on tests of force production (strength) or explosive muscular activity (power). As one representative example, a 1967 study by Costill that evaluated explosive leg strength found that untrained individuals could jump 20.9 in while elite marathon runners could jump only 13.5 in.

The low levels of muscular strength and power exhibited by most endurance athletes appear to be an adaptation to training rather than an innate trait. This can be appreciated better with the story of Lou Castagnola, a two-hour, 17-minute marathoner. In 1967 when in top shape, Lou's VO2 max was world class at 72.4 ml/kg x min while his vertical jump was only 11.5 in. Following the 1968 U.S. Olympic trials he stopped training and led a sedentary life. Three years later he was retested and it was discovered that his VO2 max had declined to 47.6 ml/kg x min, but his vertical jump actually had increased to 20.3 in. Although Lou's bone mass was not tested, it may be reasonable to assume that when in top form his bone mass was reduced, since vertical jump height has been found to be correlated with bone mass at the hip (Strong and Tucker, 2003). In the clinic, we often encounter middle-aged recreational endurance athletes who have a difficult time performing a six-inch vertical jump.

The reason for the decline in muscular strength and power that is associated with endurance exercise may be related to a variety of factors including loss of skeletal muscle, reduced levels of anabolic hormones, alteration in muscle fiber type, or energy deficit. However, the most important factor may be better understood after reading the following description of how the neuromuscular system operates.

Exercise scientists often study and discuss the neuromuscular system by compartmentalizing it into central (nervous system) and peripheral (muscular) components. The nervous system (NS) is of paramount importance in the development of muscular strength and, for our purposes, forces that ultimately act on bones. In basic terms, the NS is linked to the peripheral muscles by afferent motor nerves that innervate specific muscle fibers. This arrangement is defined as a *motor unit* (MU). Historically, MUs have been classified as being of the small and slow (type I) or large and fast (type IIb) variety, based upon a muscle cell's diameter and contraction speed. Additionally, a hybrid (type IIa) muscle fiber type with intermediate characteristics often is referred to in the scientific literature. However, it now is generally recognized by exercise scientists that muscle fibers really do not exist in discrete forms. Instead, muscle fibers at the sub cellular level exist on a continuum based upon several factors including expression of filament proteins, metabolic potential, and calcium handling characteristics. All muscles do contain both the basic slow and fast motor units but the percentage of these is unique to a particular muscle and largely genetically determined. Endurance athletes generally have a higher percentage of the slow motor units that innervate small muscle fibers, which are ideally suited for prolonged use at relatively slow velocities. Conversely, fast units have poor fatigue resistance but are capable of exerting more powerful actions.

Increases in muscle force production are achieved by different CNS mediated mechanisms. The *size principle* of muscle recruitment states that small motor units are recruited first during low intensity exercise or force requirements. Then, as force production demands are increased, and as exercise intensity is raised, larger motor units are progressively recruited. Motor units are never partially activated; they are either operational or at rest.

The other primary mechanism that increases force production is *rate coding*. Rate coding refers to the frequency at which a motor unit is activated. In general, the rate of activation of a motor unit is positively related to force production. Therefore, muscle force requirements during progressively more challenging exercise are met by the central nervous system's activation of progressively larger motor units at progressively faster firing rates. Maximal muscle force thus is achieved when both slow and fast motor units are recruited simultaneously and their rate of activation is high (fused). The ability to engage progressively larger motor units at faster rates is subject to training. Well-trained athletes are capable of activating a much higher percentage of their motor units than novices or the untrained. Major improvements in an individual's ability to generate more force can be achieved by training these nervous system pathways. This type of improvement therefore is often referred to as neuromuscular strength development, and stands in contrast to the muscular adaptations that occur in the skeletal muscles themselves, the most common being hypertrophy or enlargement.

Improvements in neuromuscular activation are achieved by exercise techniques that induce large force requirements or fast velocities or combinations of both. Please note: We did not mention efforts that induce fatigue. Fatigue in muscles can be appreciated as a reduction in force production or a decrease in velocity. Most individuals can appreciate the fatigue that results when performing a set of pull-ups or push-ups to failure. The early repetitions are executed in smooth and near effortless manner. As fatigue starts to develop, the level of effort increases and the movement speed decreases, until eventually, all movement stops and further exercise is impossible. From a neurological perspective, fatigue can be described as a reduction in both the number of motor units recruited as well as a reduction in speed at which they are operating. Therefore, if the training objective is to recruit the greatest number of motor units possible, and thereby exert greater forces on muscles and bones, exercise methods that lead to fatigue are counterproductive.

The physical characteristic that researchers often cite as being related to a muscle's strength is it's cross-sectional area (CSA) and for most individuals, especially novice athletes, there is generally a positive relationship between CSA and force production. However, it is important to realize that this correlation does not necessarily exist for either highly trained or untrained subjects. In fact, most people are familiar with individuals who have very impressive strength yet very small diameter muscles.

Muscle fibers, also known as muscle cells, are divided into smaller functional units known as *sarcomeres*. Sarcomeres contain the filament *proteins actin* and *myosin* that are responsible for muscle contraction and relaxation. At the level of the muscle, strength training has the potential to induce both *hyperplasia* (increase in muscle fiber number) and *hypertrophy* (enlargement) with hypertrophy being the more predominant consideration.

Two types of muscle fiber hypertrophy exist: sarcoplasmic and myofibrillar. *Sarcoplasmic hypertrophy* is characterized by an increase in muscle fiber size in the absence of an increase in contractile proteins, while *myofibrillar hypertrophy* occurs through increase in the volume of contractile proteins. The difference may be appreciated by the consideration of a body builder who has large muscle diameter but relatively poor strength, as compared to an Olympic style weight lifter who possesses smaller muscle mass but superior strength. Obviously, the endurance athlete considers muscle bulk that does not support improved force production capability a liability. As far as the skeleton is concerned, gains in muscle size without concomitant increases in strength are of no functional value.

The overall aim of the bone remodeling process is to achieve a skeleton that is just strong enough to withstand the largest forces that are habitually encountered by each individual athlete. Therefore, if muscular strength and power are decreased as an endurance athlete engages in exclusively low intensity endurance exercise, bone mass also will be reduced. Accordingly, for most endurance athletes, a primary cause for the progressive loss of muscular strength and power is related to the lack of recruitment of the fast motor units in training. Stated another way, you become good at what you practice. If you habitually engage in running, biking, or swimming, especially at low intensity levels and to the point of fatigue, the larger motor units never are recruited.

Although many of the specifics of bone remodeling remain undefined, *bone strain* appears to be a primary governor of the process. Strain is the term used to define the very small bending deformations that occur in bone in response to loading or stress. More specifically, if exercise-induced stresses are increased to the point at which bone strain is elevated above a certain threshold, bone formation processes are mechanically triggered. The magnitudes and frequencies of the mechanical stresses are far more important in regulating bone remodeling than the number of repetitions. To appreciate this point, a study done on rats is helpful. The experimental animals were exposed to only 10 repetitions of a high impact load at different weekly frequencies (1W, 3W, 5W, 7W) for eight weeks. Bone strength was not improved statistically in the rats exercising only one time per week yet increased by an impressive 40% in the rats performing daily exercise over those that were exercising either three or five times per week (Umemura, et al., 2008). We infer that if exercise stress levels do not induce adequate strain or are performed frequently enough, no positive remodeling will occur, regardless of how many repetitions are performed. Such is the case with greater volumes of endurance exercise; since stress levels remain constant, there is no significant increase in bone strain. Running 60 minutes versus 30 minutes does not induce greater strains on bone, only more repetitions. In a study by J.D. MacDougall and Colleagues (1992) it was reported that running up to 20 miles per week tended to increase bone mass of the lower leg but that running further (up to 75 miles/week) resulted in no further increases, but rather instead, a tendency toward reduced bone mass.

From the standpoint of long-term skeletal health, the endurance athlete needs to offset the losses of muscular and bone strength that appear as a consequence of the highly repetitious but low force demands that are characteristic of running, swimming, and cycling. To accomplish this objective, a program of exercise is needed to consistently recruit the larger motor units and thus maintain (or increase!) elevated strain levels. Interestingly enough, an individual may possess a greater amount of muscular "strength" (as defined by the amount of force that can be produced for a single repetition) prior to initiating a novel endurance-training regime than they will after getting started. In the case of an experienced athlete, strength and power often deteriorate when training volumes are increased. Unfortunately, many endurance athletes are at a loss to know what type of exercise or loading routines will reduce the likelihood of bone loss while augmenting their endurance performance.

Strength Training Considerations

1. Exercise selection
2. Parameters (frequency, intensity, volume)
3. Getting started
4. Progression
5. Integration

Exercise Selection

The primary goal of this chapter is to provide a framework for the endurance athlete to develop an exercise routine that will achieve the following objectives:

1. Decrease the likelihood of bone loss
2. Maximize general muscular strength
3. Minimize muscle hypertrophy
4. Improve endurance performance

Secondary benefits may include improved force production in sport specific movement patterns as well as reduce the potential for injury. In order to minimize excessive energy expenditure and maximize results, appropriate exercises and training parameters must be identified.

It is also important to consider that strength exercises create mainly local effects on bones (hormonal changes also occur but these are somewhat less well defined). In other words, when a muscle contracts and exerts a strain on a specific bone, only that particular bone (or part of that bone) will be influenced. Accordingly, if the primary goal of strength training is skeletal health, exercise selection must target body regions that are prone to bone loss. These locations include the spine, hip, and forearm. Furthermore, we believe that exercises should activate muscles in a manner that is consistent with function. Examples of resistance exercises that meet both criteria include:

- Dead lift
- Squat (front, back, or overhead)
- Bent row
- Lunge
- Olympic lifts (snatch, clean and jerk)

Our favorite exercises for improving total body strength are the dead lift, or what has been historically termed "the health lift," and one of the squat varieties. There now are many fine instructional videos for your review. One excellent source is the Crossfit web site (www.crossfit.com). In addition, we suggest the web site of Dan John (www.danjohn.org). Dan is a track and field coach as well as an accomplished throwing and strength athlete (American Record holder, National Weightlifting and Throwing Champion, Highland

Games competitor), lecturer, author, and academic. Although many strength and conditioning experts describe strengthening programs that require a multitude of exercises, we are in agreement with Dan when he states, in his book *Never Let Go* (2009, p. 18):

1. The body is one piece
2. There are three kinds of strength training:
    a. Putting weight overhead
    b. Picking it off the ground
    c. Carrying it for time or distance
3. All training is complementary

An extremely effective strengthening program may require performing as few as one or two exercises. For interest and variety, however, you may want to consider learning more of the basic strength exercises listed above.

Resistance Exercise Training Parameters

Examination of the cross-sectional and longitudinal research studies indicates that strength training generally results in improved bone mass and/or attenuation of age-related bone loss. However, the effect on bone can be variable and many scientific interventions have resulted in little or no effect. In fact, some studies have shown that resistance exercise actually can result in accelerated bone loss! Therefore, a thorough appreciation of what actually constitutes a successful versus unsuccessful training program is fundamental. A good example of such research was conducted in 1996 by Kerr and colleagues from the University of Western Australia. These investigators examined the skeletal response to two different training protocols: A strength group that performed three sets of eight repetitions and a muscular endurance group that performed three sets of 20 repetitions. Both groups improved their muscular strength values as determined by a *one-repetition max* weight lifting test, but only the strength group increased bone mass to a significant degree. We feel this is a very important study to consider because the featured higher repetition protocol is typical of what most endurance athletes engage in for their strength development. Unfortunately, the forces generated with this type of training appear to be inadequate for the purposes of improving bone quality. A training load that could be lifted for 20 repetitions is so small that only the small size motor units are recruited initially. As more repetitions are performed and fatigue develops, both muscular tension and bone strain is reduced. Consequently, with a training program such as this, loads on the skeleton go from relatively small to even smaller and never reach the level necessary to induce meaningful bone strain or gain.

Understanding what it takes to design and implement a successful strength routine for the skeleton requires a visit back in time to high school physics class. You may recall that force is defined by the equation mass times acceleration (F = ma). Accordingly, in order to elicit the largest forces an exercise must be performed in manner that safely utilizes large masses or fast movement speeds or a combination of both. An impressive number of studies support this exercise strategy, as reviewed by Layne and Nelson (1999). They concluded that the resistance exercise programs that have the most positive effect on bone are the trials that engage in "high-intensity" methods of training. In the sections that follow the parameters that satisfy the criteria of high intensity will be defined.

In a recent German study of postmenopausal females (Von Stengel, et al., 2007), researchers maintained a constant exercise load at 70–92.5% of the subject's one-repetition max (1RM) but altered the speed of execution. One group was instructed to exercise at a rate of four seconds for each direction of movement (concentric and eccentric) while the other group was instructed to lower the weight at the same four-second rate but perform an explosive concentric (muscle shortening) phase. After two years of study the researchers concluded that the explosively trained group lost significantly less bone mass. Also important to note was the finding that the explosively trained group experienced no significant incidence of injury or pain.

Although the optimal strength program for improving bone architecture may remain to be defined, examination of the world's strongest athletes is instructional as they generally possess the highest muscular strength as well as bone mass. Such is the case for the world record holder in the squat. In 2000, this individual at 32 years of age with a body weight of 109 kg was capable of performing a barbell squat with over 469 kg (approximately 4.3 times body weight). His lumbar spine BMD was 1.859 g/cm^2, which is 155% greater than average!

Our colleague, Professor Vladimir Zatsiorsky, in his excellent book, *Science and Practice of Strength Training* (Human Kinetics, 1995, p. 97), provides detailed training data on the distribution of weights lifted by members of the USSR Olympic team. About 85% of the team's lifts were described as being between 60–90% of the athlete's maximum competition weight (1RM). The number of repetitions per *set* in the primary lifts (snatch, clean and jerk) is two with the range being one to five. Larger-scale investigations support Zatsiorsky's findings. In 2004 Peterson and colleagues conducted a meta-analysis of the strength programs for competitive athletes at the collegiate or professional level. Their findings revealed that maximal strength gains are elicited among athletes who train at a mean training intensity of 85% of one-repetition maximum, two days per week, and with a mean training volume of eight sets.

The results just cited stand in direct contrast to most of the resistance exercise training programs recommended for endurance athletes. Standard advice is to employ low numbers of sets (one–three) with a high number of repetitions (>12–20) per set. The number of exercises per workout is generally high and often consists of isolated or single joint movements performed on machines (leg extension, leg curl, or lat pull down). In our experience, this type of protocol is of little value for the purposes of maximizing bone strength and often encourages what has been described as a segmental or "Frankenstein" like movement pattern (jerky versus coordinated or athletic in nature). Additionally, because these protocols generally are performed to exhaustion, injury risk may be elevated and *recovery* may be prolonged. Lastly, sets performed in this range of repetitions have been shown to induce muscle hypertrophy, presumably of the sarcoplasmic variety, that results in non-functional body mass.

Strength needs to be defined as either being *absolute* or *relative.* Absolute strength is the term used to describe the amount of weight an athlete can lift independent of her or his size, whereas relative strength is the amount of weight an athlete can lift compared to body mass. In endurance competition, the primary resistance that must be moved is the athlete's own body weight. From this central observation, it becomes obvious that it is essential to train for relative strength to body mass, rather than absolute strength per se. However, it is important to realize that increases in an athlete's absolute strength are associated with improvements in their relative strength (provided that body mass is not also increased). Maximal absolute strength levels with minimal body mass will produce optimal performance in activities such as cycling, swimming, or rowing. The basic degree of hypertrophy an individual achieves with resistance exercise is multifactorial and influenced by gender, age, hormone levels, and nutritional status, etc. Maximal hypertrophy is apparently a consequence of tension, vascular (ischemia) perturbation, and the degradation of protein elements. Strength training, versus body building or hypertrophy training, specializes in the development of tension without inducing severe ischemia or the degradation of contractile proteins, minimizing the likelihood of building muscle mass that does not support increased force production.

In contrast to body builders, strength athletes train with a limited number of exercises, done in multiple sets of one to six repetitions per set. Rest periods between sets are prolonged to allow for short-term recovery to be achieved. Since fatigue leads to reductions in motor unit recruitment, and thus force production, training to the point of muscular exhaustion is unusual. Strength athletes do not train to fail, they train to succeed. Training occurs frequently, often daily, sometimes multiple times per day. Volume and intensity are varied frequently as consistency is known to cause stagnation. As strength levels increase, training overload is created by adding more weight rather than additional repetitions.

Many endurance athletes have been conditioned to believe that strength training will at best not improve performance and at worst diminish it. However, numerous studies now confirm that a well-designed strength program will improve not only bone mass but endurance performance as well (Table 1.1).

Table 1.1 Comparison of strength versus endurance training protocols

Protocol	Frequency/ Week	Exercises/ Workout	Sets/ Exercise	Reps/ Set	Rest
Endurance	Low (1–3)	High (>6)	Low (1–3)	>12–20	1–3 min
Strength	High (>3)	Low (2)	High (>4)	<6	>3 min

An excellent perspective on resistance training for running performance is provided by Linda Yamamoto and colleagues (2008): "The effects of resistance training on endurance performance among highly trained runners: a systematic review." The authors conclude that both running performance and running economy can be expected to improve as a result of a well-planned training program that includes concurrent running and strength training components.

Perhaps the most compelling individual study that has been performed to date was that of Paavolainen and colleagues (1999). These researchers divided a group of highly trained runners that were averaging 75 running miles per week. One group continued their typical training, which consisted of a traditional balance of endurance, speed, and strength workouts, while the other group reduced running mileage to 50 miles per week and started a program of short sprints, plyometric jumps (with and without weights), and strength exercises performed with rapid speeds. Following nine weeks of training, the traditional volume group showed increases in both maximal oxygen consumption and *lactate* thresholds; as a result they could work longer and harder than they could previously, but running speeds or 5 km performances were unchanged. Conversely, the experimental group did not show any improvement in the laboratory measures but were able to run significantly faster and improved their 5 km performance by nearly 30 seconds.

When endurance athletes question whether training with exclusively heavy loads and minimal numbers of exercises can influence performance in addition to improving bone mass, we like to cite the results of a recent study performed by Storen and colleagues (2008). In this study, 17 male and female runners were divided into two treatment groups: an experimental group that participated in an eight-week program of strength training, and a control group that continued their habitual running program. The strength training protocol required the subjects to perform four sets of partial squats (free weights) using a 4RM load. When a subject could complete a set with five repetitions, 2.5 kg were added to the next set. Each set of squats was separated by three minutes of rest, and the training frequency was three times per week. The results were impressive and consistent with what we anticipate in the athletes that we train. Specifically, significant improvements in 1RM ½ squat (33.2%), rate of force development (26%), running economy (5%), and time to exhaustion at maximal *aerobic* speed (21.3%) were recorded in the strength trained group, while there was no significant changes in the controls.

Getting Started

If you have never participated in a strength-training program, we recommend a period of time dedicated to learning proper technique as well as to allow for various body tissues (muscle, tendon, bone) to adapt to new mechanical loads. We advise cautious progression, since the amount of weight you can lift will increase quickly as a result of learning (central or neural factors) and may supersede the adaptation capability of your connective tissues (tendons).

To decrease the likelihood of sustaining an overuse injury (tendonitis) during the developmental stages of a strength program, we recommend 8–12 weeks of training with loads less than or equal to 65% of the one-repetition maximum (RM) load. This is generally the amount of weight that could be lifted to failure for 15 repetitions (see Table 1.2). For example, consider performing sets of non-fatiguing repetitions with a 65% 1RM load for your selected exercises two–four times per week. Controlled movements with meticulous exercise technique should be the focus during this time. Movement speed should be dictated by control but may be variable in order to facilitate learning. To start, we generally recommend three–four seconds for each of the concentric and eccentric phases. Additionally, we encourage the use of a minimalist shoe without excessive heel height or arch support. We discourage the use of mirrors for feedback and even advocate that some repetitions should be performed with eyes closed in order to better facilitate stability, balance, and the development of new motor skills. Sample workouts for a select exercise during the developmental stage of a resistance exercise program may include:

Table 1.2 Sample workouts
Workout 1: 4 sets of 4–6 repetitions
Workout 2: 3 sets of 6–8 repetitions
Workout 3: 2 sets of 8–10 repetitions

%1RM	Reps
100	1
95	2
90	4
85	6
80	8
75	10
70	12
65	15

Weight training loads often are described as a percentage of the one-repetition maximum (1RM). An individual's 1RM load is the amount of weight that could actually or theoretically be lifted only one time. Accordingly, the 6RM load is the maximal amount of weight that could be lifted exactly six times. This table is to be considered only a general guideline in estimating training loads as the relationship between %1RM and maximal repetitions is variable among individuals as well as exercises.

Following the completion of this early adaptation phase, precision technique for all lifts must be established. Specific attention should be paid to the position of the spine as well as the maintenance of a "tight" feeling of the abdominals and trunk musculature during the execution of all lifts. Additionally, adequate range of motion must be established to ensure that movements are performed in a non-compensatory manner. All individuals, especially those new to strength training, should consider the consultation of a physical therapist, certified athletic trainer, or strength and conditioning professional to ensure that adequate mobility and proper execution are achieved.

As a basic screening procedure attempt the following self-administered test: Stand less than 2 inches from a wall; head level with eyes looking straight ahead; palms facing the wall (away from you). Slowly descend into a squat position while maintaining the head in a horizontal position. Performing this test in front of a wall ensures that the knee is not traveling too far in front of the foot and that the spinal curves are relatively well maintained. The level to which you can descend with good balance and control represents the bottom of the range for which you can safely perform lifts such as the deadlift or squat. If you attempt this same procedure with the arms overhead it will indicate the range within which you can safely descend in the overhead squat. If your range of motion is found to be limited (which often is the case for endurance athletes we work with) and you cannot achieve a position in which your thigh is parallel to the floor, consider consulting a movement specialist who can assist you with range of motion restoration, or assist you with a modification of the exercise. Some athletes may want to consider using a Hex Deadlift Bar or a Super Deadlift Bar (Power Systems, Inc.) as this may offer certain biomechanical advantages over a conventional straight bar. For general screening purposes Physical Therapist Gray Cook (2006) has published two excellent articles that detail seven functional movement tests that we utilize for our athletes prior to engaging in resistance exercise or sport participation.

Low back pain is a very common problem in modern societies. Perhaps the greatest risk factor for the development of pain is the tremendous amount of sitting that most jobs entail. This habit often is problematic especially in the athletic population, since fatigue following training appears to exaggerate poor sitting posture. Prolonged slouched sitting leads to a gradual loss of the inward curve in the lower back (lordosis) and back bending capability. As backward bending (extension) becomes more limited, the spine becomes more vulnerable as the intervertebral disc and supporting ligamentous structures are rendered unstable. Often, an acute exacerbation of pain comes for "no apparent reason" but is mistakenly blamed on the trivial task during which the pain developed (bending over to pick up a pencil, taking out the trash).

In order to protect the lower back while engaged in strength training several key elements should be considered. First and foremost, the lordosis or inward curve of the back must be maintained. Robin

McKenzie, a world-renowned physical therapist from New Zealand, recommends performing back bending movements (extension exercise) immediately prior to and following any strenuous activities such as weight lifting. This can be done in the standing position but is perhaps more effectively done in the prone (lying face down) position. Place your palms on the floor as if you were going to perform a standard push-up. Straighten your elbows, but allow your lower back to remain relaxed and on the floor. At the top of the movement pause for two to three seconds to allow for complete relaxation of the lower back. This restores the maximal back bending mobility in the spine that is frequently lost after slouched sitting. Most adults should be able to easily achieve an elbow lock while hips remain in contact with the floor. If tightness or pain is experienced in the lower back region with this maneuver, a loss of spinal mobility (dysfunction) has occurred. This condition often is improved with the consistent application of the exercise throughout the day. In general, we recommend six to 10 repetitions per session, three to five sessions per day, for as many days as it takes to eliminate the tightness. Several weeks of work may be needed in cases of long-standing mobility loss. Following the resolution of tightness, this exercise should be practiced at least once daily, preferably before and/or immediately following weight training or periods of sustained forward bending, including cycling or rowing.

We often recommend cyclists and rowers read a magazine or newspaper for five to 15 minutes in the prone position (propped up on elbows) immediately following prolonged training sessions. This brief rest period ensures that the loss of spinal extension is fully restored, and reduces the likelihood of an acute attack of lower back pain. Additionally, use of a lumbar support to maintain the lordosis should be standard practice for all individuals who engage in prolonged sitting. For further assistance with the management of lower back or neck pain we recommend that you contact the McKenzie Institute International.

Progression

Transition from the early *adaptation* phase to an increased loading level should be gradual rather than abrupt. For endurance athletes and others interested in training for bone acquisition or minimizing bone loss, increasing weight to at least the 85% of 1RM level is indicated. This loading level will correlate approximately with a weight that can be lifted a maximum of six times (6RM) prior to failure. Again, endurance athletes should rarely (or never) perform strength exercises to failure. Instead, multiple sets of an exercise should be performed in a manner that enables the athlete to develop maximal tension during the lift without allowing muscle failure to occur. For example, a variety of daily strength sessions for an individual with a 6RM dead lift of 185 lbs and a 6RM bent row of 120 lbs may look like this:

Workout 1
Dead lift: 4 sets of 3–5 repetitions at 185 lbs

Workout 2
Bent row: 4 sets of 3–5 repetitions at 120 lbs

Workout 3
Dead lift: 2 sets of 3–5 repetitions at 185 lbs
Bent row: 2 sets of 3–5 repetitions at 120 lbs

Workout 4
Dead lift: 6 sets (2, 4, 6, 2, 4, 6 repetitions/set) at 175 lbs

Workout 5
Bent row:
1 set of 2–3 repetitions of 135 lbs
1 set of 2–3 repetitions of 155 lbs
1 set of 2–3 repetitions of 175 lbs
1 set of 2–3 repetitions of 195 lbs

We generally have described workouts with fewer sets than what would be considered typical for the strength specialist. Based upon the tenets of bone remodeling, large volumes of exercise do not appear necessary to maximize bone acquisition or minimize bone loss. The frequency and intensity of the loading rather than volume of exercise appear to be far more important determinants of skeletal adaptation. This point was illustrated in one recent study, (Kato, et al., 2006) as *bone mineral density* (BMD) at both the hip and lumbar spine were shown to increase significantly in female subjects performing only 10 maximal vertical jumps three times per week.

The rate of strength development appears to be highly variable, but related chiefly to the volume or intensity of the endurance athlete's sport specific demands or competitive season. Consequently, strength training may take a higher or lower priority during certain times of the year. Make periodic changes in your training weights as strength levels improve. These adjustments need not be an overly formal process, but note when you are capable of achieving over six repetitions with a former 6RM value. Once this level is reached, we recommend increasing your training loads rather than adding more sets or repetitions. Decreases in strength from habitual levels indicate that additional rest or recovery from endurance training is needed or that an over-reaching state is being approached. Remember that during times of demanding endurance training, your resistance exercise should be thought of as a means of reducing the likelihood of losing strength and bone mass; not necessarily a time for increasing strength. During phases of the year in which endurance volumes are lowest or when "A" priority events are in the distant future are ideal periods to dedicate toward improving basic strength. Think of these times as opportunities to make deposits in your bone bank that you may need to rely on in the future.

Integration

One question that we are consistently asked is how to integrate strength exercise into an endurance athlete's training plan; concerns about time constraint and recovery abound. Because an effective session of bone building exercise may be as brief as the time required to perform 10 maximal vertical jumps or two sets of resistance exercise, the actual time necessary to prevent bone loss is small. However, the time spent commuting to a gym often make strength sessions difficult to incorporate. For busy endurance athletes interested in pursuing a regular program of strength training, we strongly encourage the acquisition of some basic home gym equipment. All that is required is a quality set of free weights (barbell and plates) and possibly a rack or stand. The amount of weight required is of course individual, but for most male and female endurance athletes, a barbell set with 225 lbs and 185 lbs respectively, is sufficient. Other pieces of relatively inexpensive supplemental home equipment include kettlebells, a pull up bar, and a sturdy box (for vertical jumps).

Exercise Order

Most scientific studies demonstrate that if endurance exercise precedes strength exercise, the quality of the strength sessions will be diminished for up to eight hours. This pattern may be related to a variety of factors including dehydration, hormonal perturbations, or central/peripheral fatigue. Conversely, strength exercises performed prior to endurance training sessions appear to have little or no detrimental effect on endurance performance. We feel this is especially

Table 1.3 Endurance athlete's guide to bone health, strength program overview

Frequency	Exercises per workout	Intensity % of 1RM	Sets/ Exercise	Repetitions/ Set	Rest between sets
2–4 Xs/ week	1–3	75–90	2–6	2–6	> 2 min

true if the strength session is performed without inducing muscle failure. If strength sessions are of the high volume fatigue inducing nature, delayed recovery is inevitable and endurance performance may be limited for both the short and long term (see Table 1.3).

A recent scientific study illustrated very convincingly that training to muscular failure is not only unnecessary, but may be detrimental to strength and endurance performance. In 2009, researchers from Spain evaluated the efficacy of an eight-week program of resistance training to failure versus not training to failure at both moderate and low volumes for increasing upper body strength and power. Forty-three trained male rowers were matched and randomly assigned to four groups that performed the same endurance training but differed on their resistance training regime: four exercises leading to repetition failure (4RF), four exercises not leading to failure (4NRF), two exercises not to failure (2NRF) and a control group (C). The researchers concluded that during an eight-week concurrent strength- and endurance-training program using a moderate number of repetitions not to failure provides a favorable environment for achieving greater enhancements in strength, muscle power, and rowing performance when compared with higher training volumes or repetitions to failure in experienced oarsman.

Summary

Participation in endurance exercise is associated with reduced muscular strength and power production presumably related to the habitual recruitment of slow motor units. A well-planned program of resistance exercise has the potential to maintain or improve muscular strength, bone mass, and endurance performance.

The cornerstone of an endurance athlete's strength routine should be the consistent performance of a small number of exercises that provide loading to the skeletal regions that are most prone to bone loss (spine, hip, and forearm). In order to minimize the likelihood of prolonged recovery and/or muscle hypertrophy, avoid training to the point of muscular exhaustion. Acquisition of basic exercise equipment for the home will ensure consistency in the program as well as eliminate both gym fees and travel time.

The intensity level demonstrated to be necessary to achieve the greatest improvements in muscular and thus bone strength is in the order of 75–90% of the 1RM. This is generally the amount of weight that can be lifted a maximum of six times. The exercise parameters that appear to be of the greatest importance for muscle and bone strength are the frequency and intensity of loading. In general we would suggest performing more than two resistance-training sessions per week throughout the year. For endurance specialists the sets and repetitions of your strength routine need not be overly formal or regimented. In order to prevent bone loss and preserve muscular strength while engaged in primarily endurance based exercise, the most important consideration is to load your skeleton consistently with forces that are adequate to create bone strains that are well beyond those that are consistent with endurance training.

To maximize your strength gains we generally recommend the performance of strength exercises prior to endurance training. However, we have had excellent results in decreasing the sensation of "heavy legs" in certain athletes by having them perform two to three sets of strengthening exercises immediately following an endurance exercise session. Other techniques that can serve a similar purpose include the performance of a six to 10 vertical jumps (jumping up to an elevated surface rather than the reverse) or the performance of one to two sets of "swings" with a kettlebell.

For a comprehensive coverage of resistance exercise and strength training, we highly recommend a book by our colleague Dr. Vladimir Zatsiorsky, *Science and Practice of Strength Training* (Human Kinetics, 1995). For any endurance athlete interested in pursuing a program of body building type training for the purposes of improving body composition or increasing muscular size, we suggest Pavel Tsatsouline's *Beyond Bodybuilding* (Dragon Door Publications, 2005). For a recent scientific review article on the subject of strength training and bone mass, we refer you to the work of Nguyen and colleagues (2008).

REFERENCES

Cook G, Burton L, Hoogenboom B (2006) Pre-participation screening: the use of fundamental movements as an assessment of function, part 1. *North American Journal of Sports Physical Therapy* 1(2):62–72.

Cook G, Burton L, Hoogenboom B (2006) Pre-participation screening: the use of fundamental movements as an assessment of function, part 2. *North American Journal of Sports Physical Therapy* 1(3):132–139.

Costill DL (1967) The relationship between selected physiologic variables and distance running performance. *Journal of Sports Medicine and Physical Fitness* 7:61–66.

John DA (2009) *Never Let Go A Philosophy of Lifting, Living, and Learning.* Aptos, CA: On Target Publications.

Kato T, Terashima T, Hatanaka Y, Honda A, Umemura Y (2006) Effects of low-repetition jump training on bone mineral density in young women. *Journal of Applied Physiology* 100(3):839–843.

Kerr D, Morton A, Dick I, Prince R (1996) Exercise effects on bone mass in postmenopausal women are site-specific and load-dependent. *Journal of Bone and Mineral Research* 11(2):218–225.

Layne JE, Nelson ME (1999) The effects of progressive resistance training on bone density: a review. *Medicine and Science in Sports and Exercise* 31(1):25–30.

lzquierdo-Gabarren M, Gonzalez de Txabarri Exposito R, Garcia-Pallares J, Sanchez- Medina L, Saez de Villarreal ES, lzquierdo M (2009) Concurrent endurance and strength training not to failure optimizes performance gains. *Medicine and Science in Sports and Exercise* 42(6):1191–1199.

MacDougall J, Webber C, Martin J, Ormerod S, Chesley A, Yonglai E, Gordon C, Blimkie J (1992) Relationship among running mileage, bone density, and serum testosterone in male runners. *Journal of Applied Physiology* 73(3):1165–1170.

Nguyen VH, Loethen JMA, LaFontaine T (2008) Resistance training and dietary supplementation for persons with reduced bone mineral density. *Strength & Conditioning Journal* 30(5):28–31.

Paavolainen L, Kakkinen K, Hammalainen I, Nummela A, Rusko H (1999) Explosive-strength training improves 5-km running time by improving running economy and muscle power. *Journal of Applied Physiology* 86(5):1527–1533.

Peterson MD, Rhea MR, Alvar BA (2004) Maximizing strength development in athletes: a meta-analysis to determine the dose-response relationship. *Journal of Strength and Conditioning Research* 18(2):377–382.

Storen O, Helgerud E, Stoa E, Hoff J (2008) Maximal strength training improves running economy in distance runners. *Medicine and Science in Sports and Exercise* 40(6):1087–1092.

Strong J, Tucker L (2003) Vertical jump height is predictive of hip bone mineral density in middle-aged women. *Medicine and Science in Sports and Exercise* 35(5):S21.

Tsatsouline P (2005) *Beyond Bodybuilding.* St. Paul, MN: Dragon Door Publications.

Tucci JT, Carpenter DM, Pollock ML, Graves JE, Leggett SH (1992) Effect of reduced frequency of training and detraining on lumbar extension strength. *Spine* 17:1479–1501.

Umemura Y, Nagasawa, Honda A, Singh R (2008) High-impact exercise frequency per week or day for osteogenic response in rats. *Journal of Bone Mineral Metab*olism 26(5):456–460.

Von Stengel S, Kemmler W, Kalender WA, Engelke K, Lauber D (2007) Differential effects of strength versus power training on bone mineral density in postmenopausal women: a 2-year longitudinal study. *British Journal of Sports Medicine* 41(10):649–655.

Yamamoto L, Lopez R, Klau J, Casa D, Kraemer W, Maresh C (2008) The effects of resistance training on endurance distance running performance among highly trained runners: a systematic review. *Journal of Strength and Conditioning Research* 22(6):2036–2044.

Zatsiorsky V (1995) *Science and Practice of Strength Training.* Champaign, IL: Human Kinetics.

CHAPTER TWO

Nutrition

Most endurance athletes understand the fundamental truth that food is fuel. However, for those interested in maximizing physical performance and maintaining skeletal health, a more thorough understanding of exercise-nutrition interactions is necessary. There is now abundant evidence that many endurance athletes exist in a chronically energy deficient state. Such energy deficits may be created by either excessive exercise expenditure or through inadequate dietary intake, and commonly a combination of both. When energy deficit exists, bone mass and strength are reduced. Hormonal and nutritionally mediated pathways, often in interaction, can lead to serious bone loss. Therefore, rule number one regarding endurance exercise and bone is that energy balance needs to be maintained.

In 2000, researchers Cathy Zanker and Ian Swaine evaluated eight well-trained male distance runners (mean age 25.1 years) under experimental training conditions in which energy balance was either maintained or negative (50% energy deficit). According to the protocol for the research, the athletes ran for 60 minutes on a treadmill during each of three consecutive days. The 60-minute runs were divided into four 15-minute intervals, each of which comprised three five-minute periods of running at intensities equivalent to 65%, 75%, and 85% of each subject's maximal oxygen consumption. Results showed that during the energy deficient state there were reductions of 15% and 17%, respectively, in the blood concentrations of P1NP (a marker of bone formation, the full name of which is type 1 procollagen with an NH_2 terminal unit) and IGF-1 (an important growth factor for bone); in contrast, the concentrations of these bone-building compounds were stable during the three days of exercise in which energy balance was maintained.

Endurance athletes place unique demands on their bodies, requiring adequate food energy for development, maintenance, and repair of physiologic systems. Foods that we eat are ingested as large macronutrient complexes known as carbohydrates, fats, and proteins. These large molecules are digested into smaller particles (sugars, fatty acids, amino acids) that can be absorbed through the intestinal wall and delivered to either working muscles or storage. Food energy is stored in the form of glucose or triglycerides in the liver, muscle, and adipose tissues (fat). During exercise, these fuels are delivered to the muscle cell mitochondria, where molecules of *adenosine triphosphate* (ATP) are produced. ATP is the body's terminal source of energy for muscular contractions.

Protein can serve as an energy source in metabolism, but carbohydrate and fat are the body's preferred fuel sources. Both carbohydrate and fat are involved in supplying energy, although their individual contributions vary under different circumstances. Which of these common fuels is used depends on multiple factors including exercise intensity and duration. In general, during low to moderate intensity exercise (< 60% VO2 max), fatty acids supply a large percentage of the substrate; however, as exercise intensity is increased (>75% VO2 max), carbohydrate becomes the predominant fuel source.

Historically, scientists interested in exercise-nutrition interactions correlated muscle glycogen levels with performance and provided convincing evidence that increased carbohydrate availability improved performance. In 1971 Karlsson and Saltin found that times in a 30 km crosscountry race were best when the pre-race muscle glycogen stores were maximized to a range of 440 g with a carbohydrate loading protocol, whereas times were 12 minutes slower when runners followed a high protein-fat diet resulting in muscle glycogen levels in the 230 g range. Similarly, in 1984 Bebb and colleagues showed that subjects who engaged in carbohydrate loading for three days were able to run 12% longer at 70% VO2 max than could those who followed normal diets.

Endogenous carbohydrate storage is limited relative to the storage of fat. Most studies of exercise energy metabolism reveal that a trained athlete can perform at a high intensity level (70–85% VO2 max) for a period of approximately two hours. After that time, carbohydrate levels appear to decline to a level that limits performance. This drop is described by scientists as exercise-induced hypoglycemia, or by athletes as "bonking" or "hitting the wall." If exercise duration continues, such as during an ultramarathon running event or a century (100 mile) bike ride, the percentage of fat metabolism is increased. Dr. David Costill of Ball State University, who performed some of the classic research in the field of endurance fuel utilization, has reported that the contribution of fat utilization is increased from 39% to 65% over two hours of continuous running at 65% of VO2 max (1970).

Carbohydrate metabolism includes the breakdown of starches and sugars into the subunit glucose. Glucose is stored in the liver and muscle as glycogen. A well-trained individual may store twice the amount of glycogen as a person who does not exercise. In general, liver glycogen stores are in the range of 100 g, while muscle storage is on the order of 300–800 g. Liver glycogen is utilized at a rate of approximately 10 g per hour during resting conditions and may be released and consumed by muscles at a rate of 50–60 g per hour during exercise.

To offset the reduction in muscle and liver glycogen associated with endurance exercise, sports nutritionists historically have recommended that athletes consume a diet rich in carbohydrates. A high-carbohydrate diet generally is considered one in which carbohydrate intake provides at least 60% of the total energy intake. However, this may not be an ideal recommendation for either performance or bone health. First and foremost, we find that certain athletes have a difficult time balancing their exercise expenditure when consuming mainly carbohydrate-based fare. Among others, Hawley and colleagues (1995) have shown that an athlete's appetite is a poor indicator of the caloric requirements needed to balance exercise expenditure. This finding is in sharp contrast to effects of a diet-induced energy deficit, which is known to lead to an increase in appetite and preoccupation with food. Because many carbohydrate foods are high in volume and low in calories, an athlete's appetite may be satisfied prior to restoration of energy-balance.

Horvath and colleagues (2000) reported that when recreational male and female runners were allowed to eat as much as they desired from a carbohydrate rich meal plan, overall energy balance was not maintained. In another example, Onywera and colleagues (2004) detailed the dietary patterns of a group of elite Kenyan distance runners and found that, when eating a diet composed of 76.5% carbohydrate and 13.4% fat, the runners developed an energy deficit of approximately 600 kcal per day. When the subjects in the Horvath study increased their overall energy intake by increasing their fat intake from 17% to 31%, their running performance at 80% VO2 max improved by an impressive 18%. Energy balance was maintained!

Although many of our athletes have been conditioned to believe that a high-carbohydrate meal plan is optimal, it is important to realize that there is no one-size-fits-all nutritional approach. In fact, many successful athletes have adapted well to a meal plan of moderate carbohydrate intake with a greater reliance on fat for energy. Researchers investigating the topic report that in many cases a more fat-dependent strategy may lead to better energy balance, reductions in injury, increases in bone mass, and even improved performance.

In the *Journal of the International Society of Sports Nutrition*, Kristen Gerlach and her colleagues from the University of Buffalo monitored 86 female runners for over a year and discovered that low fat intake was the single best dietary predictor of injury risk. In fact, their analysis revealed that fat intake (or the lack thereof!) correctly identified 64% of future injuries.

Historically, the sports nutrition literature has promoted the performance benefits of consuming carbohydrates prior to exercise. However, it is becoming more evident that chronic consumption of high carbohydrate foods is not necessary for maintenance or restoration of glycogen stores. With moderate carbohydrate intake (seven to ten g/kg body mass per day) muscle glycogen stores can be replenished to satisfactory levels within 24 hours. Additionally, little performance advantage appears to be gained by attempting to "top off the tank" by overloading with carbohydrates prior to training or competition.

Although pre-exercise muscle glycogen levels are important for performance, a greater concern is the maintenance of adequate blood glucose levels during exercise. This shift in focus is especially important for events lasting longer than 90–120 minutes. The prevention of hypoglycemia during prolonged exercise can be achieved in ways other than by consuming a primarily high carbohydrate diet. Specifically, athletes may consume a carbohydrate-rich meal several hours prior to exercise and/or utilize supplementing carbohydrate during exercise.

Here is an example of how such nutritional patterns can support high performance: A world-class lightweight rower was evaluated over a two-month training period as he was preparing for the 1995 world rowing championships. The subject trained for approximately 70 minutes per day at variable intensities to simulate race conditions. Caloric expenditures (based upon heart rate response and estimation from specific activity) were estimated at 4,125 kcal/day. A three-day diet survey revealed that he maintained caloric balance, as intake was determined to be 4,088 kcal/day. Analysis of macronutrient intake revealed protein, carbohydrate, and fat made up 19%, 51%, and 30% of his caloric intake, respectively. During and after training, the subject consumed two separate carbohydrate supplements that added a total of 218 g of carbohydrate per day. This level of supplementation was able to maintain the subject's blood glucose concentration at normal levels following recovery from exercise. Despite consuming carbohydrates at a lower than recommended maintenance level, this athlete won three world championship gold medals (Xia G, et al., 2001).

Additionally, there are several studies that suggest athletes actually perform better on a high fat diet. In 2005, Robins and colleagues investigated the response of two highly trained male rowers to both a high fat diet (60% fat, 30% CHO, 10% protein) and a high carbohydrate diet (20% fat, 70% CHO, 10% protein). Each of the dietary trials lasted 14 days and was followed by an ultra distance rowing trial performed at 60% VO2 max (two hours on and two off, for 24 hours). The results demonstrated that both subjects were able to row a greater distance (with a concomitant reduced heart rate, volume of oxygen uptake, and respiratory exchange ratio) following the high fat as opposed to high carbohydrate diet. Additional studies that have reported similar findings include Phinney, et al., 1983; Lambert, et al., 1994; Muio, et al., 1994; and Hoppeler, et al., 1999.

Just as there has been interest in the use of higher fat diets for endurance athletes, there also has been strong support for performance improvement in experimental animal studies. Miller and colleagues (1984) have demonstrated improvements as great as 33% in rats within only five weeks of adapting to a high fat diet. Dietary fats can serve as a nearly inexhaustible substrate for energy production, since even the leanest of athletes can store enough fat to produce energy for days. Along with many of the carbohydrates that we consume, dietary fats are digested, absorbed, and stored as triglycerides located in adipose, liver, and muscle tissues. Stored triglycerides are made available for energy production during exercise, at which time they undergo hydrolysis (breakdown) into simpler constituents, free fatty acids (FFA), and glycerol. Free fatty acids are transported in the blood to the muscle cell mitochondria, where ATP is formed and made available to energize muscular contractions.

The studies that have been performed to date indicate that endurance athletes have the capacity to adapt equally well to a variety of diets. In fact, studies of evolutionary human nutrition reveal that carbohydrate intake was primarily opportunistic and many populations have survived on protein and fat to the near exclusion of carbohydrate. The Masai tribesman of Africa (who eat meat, blood, and milk of their cattle) and the Arctic Inuit (who consume reindeer meat and seal blubber) are classic examples.

For more information on this topic we recommend Stephen Phinney's (2004) article "Ketogenic diets and physical performance" published in *Nutrition and Metabolism*). Dr. Phinney provides an excellent historical perspective on how the contemporary recommendation that endurance athletes consume a primarily carbohydrate based diet evolved. In addition, he details the stories of Lt. Frederick Schwatka and Vilhjalmur Stefansson, both of whom had the opportunity to live with Inuit people and eat a traditional Inuit diet for extended periods. The diet was essentially devoid of carbohydrate and consisted of approximately 15–25% protein and 85% fat. In a journal entry, Schwatka revealed that his stamina remained intact as he and an Inuit companion walked 65 miles in less than 48 hours to make a scheduled rendezvous with a whaling ship. The key features of Phinney's article include three requirements needed for adaptation to a low carbohydrate regime. This unusual research helps us to appreciate that humans have the capacity to adapt to a variety of dietary patterns and that certain individuals may in fact be better served by a diet that is not entirely carbohydrate focused.

In a landmark study performed in the laboratory of Tim Noakes, MD, doctoral student Julia Goedecke demonstrated that after an overnight fast there is great variability in the metabolism both at rest and during exercise of equally performing recreational cyclists. At rest, the percentage of fat metabolized was normally distributed, varying from 25% to 100%. During a graduated exercise protocol at 25%, 50%, and 70% of peak work rate, this normal distribution was maintained but shifted to the right, indicating that carbohydrate metabolism increased commensurate with exercise intensity. At the 70% workload, some individuals derived as much as 40% of their energy from fat while others derived 100% of their energy from carbohydrate (Goedecke, et al., 2000). The importance of this study cannot be overstated, as it demonstrates the highly individual patterns by which athletes metabolize stored energy supplies. Athletes with a predisposition for fat metabolism are likely to require less carbohydrate supplementation during prolonged exercise and less carbohydrate replenishment following exercise as compared to an athlete that preferentially metabolizes carbohydrate. The determinants of these differences in energy utilization patterns remain unknown. They may be genetically influenced or conditioned by long-term patterns of diet and exercise. Indeed, it is possible that both factors are involved, with even the patterns of interaction differing among individuals.

Despite the relatively small contribution of protein to energy metabolism, prolonged endurance exercise has been associated with significant increases in protein turnover (degradation and synthesis). However, these findings have been contradictory and appear to be related to measurement techniques utilized by researchers, as well as whether carbohydrate availability and total energy availability were controlled. In general, if energy availability, specifically carbohydrate levels, is maintained, protein stores and performance are preserved. However, when energy balance is negative and when carbohydrate levels decline, protein degradation ensues (Koopman, et al., 2004).

Independent of adequate carbohydrate availability, specific amino acids (those with branched chains in their molecular structures) are required for the metabolism of both carbohydrate and fat. During exercise these *branched chain amino acids* are removed from protein stores. Although supplementation with protein during exercise has not been demonstrated convincingly to improve performance, some studies have revealed that muscle damage may be decreased. A protective effect of this sort appears to be especially true in the case of untrained subjects or in trained subjects who are increasing exercise volume or intensity.

In 2007 Greer and colleagues evaluated markers of muscle damage following a 90-minute cycling bout at 55% VO2 max in untrained male volunteers. Subjects consumed either a 200 kcal carbohydrate beverage, a beverage containing isocaloric branched chain amino acids, or a non-caloric placebo beverage. Creatine kinase (CK), lactate dehydrogenase (LDH), leg strength, and muscle soreness were assessed before and immediately following exercise as well as at three points (4, 24, and 48 hours) after exercise. Results demonstrated that CK activity was significantly lower after the BCAA (Branched Chain Amino Acid) trial than the placebo trial at all points post-exercise, as well as lower than the carbohydrate beverage at 24 hours post-exercise. CK was lower in the carbohydrate trial at the 24- and 48-hour time points than in the placebo trial. LDH activity was lower in the BCAA trial at four hours than in the placebo trial. Compared with the carbohydrate and placebo trials, ratings of muscle soreness were lower at 24 hours and leg strength was higher at 48 hours after the BCAA trial.

Summary

Collectively, the above findings suggest that optimal endurance nutrition may be individually unique and dependent on each particular athlete's genetic variability, historical consumption, and training status, as well as the availability of food resources. In summary, we offer the following key points:

- Adequate energy availability must be maintained in order to preserve normal hormonal and skeletal health.
- Diet composition with respect to carbohydrate and fat may be unique to the individual and related to multiple factors.

- Maintenance of blood glucose levels during exercise is important for performance as well as to prevent the degradation of protein (muscle) stores.

- Diets that are primarily carbohydrate based may make it difficult for athletes to meet energy demands and result in an energy deficit.

- Increasing dietary fat may reduce energy deficit, decrease injury risk, and/or improve performance.

- Consider slight deficits in energy balance as possible causes of poor performance or failure to improve.

- Suspect overt energy deficit in cases of menstrual cycle disturbance, stress fracture, or overtraining syndrome.

- Endurance athletes must understand how to calculate their exercise expenditure and be able to counter this with sound nutritional intake. Guidelines for these considerations will be detailed in subsequent chapters.

REFERENCES

Bebb J, Brewer J, Patton A, Williams C (1984) Endurance running and the influence of diet on fluid intake. *Journal of Sport Sciences* 2:198–199.

Costill D (1970) Metabolic responses during distance running. *Journal of Applied Physiology* 28:251–255.

Gerlach K, Burton H, Dorn J, Leddy J, Horvath P (2008) Fat intake and injury in female runners. *Journal of the International Society of Sports Nutrition* 5:1. Complete electronic version: http://www.jissn.com/content/5/1/1.

Goedecke JH, St. Clair Gibson A, Grobler L, Collins M, Noakes T, Lambert E (2000) Determinants of the variability in respiratory exchange ratio at rest and during exercise in trained athletes. *American Journal of Physiology* 5:1.

Greer B, Woodard J, White J, Arquello E, Haymes E (2007) Branched-chain amino acid supplementation and indicators of muscle damage after endurance exercise. *International Journal of Sports Nutrition and Exercise Metabolism* 17(6):595–607.

Hawley J, Dennis S, Lindsay F, Noakes T (1995) Nutritional practices of athletes: are they sub-optimal? *Journal of Sport Sciences* 13:S75–81.

Hoppeler H, Billeter R, Horvath P, Leddy J, Pendergast D (1999) Muscle structure with low and high fat diets in well trained endurance runners. *International Journal of Sports Medicine* 20:522–526.

Horvath P, Eagen C, Ryer-Calvin S, Pendergast DR (2000) The effects of varying dietary fat on the nutrient intake in male and female runners. *Journal of the American College of Nutrition* 19(1):42–51, 52–60.

Karlsson J, Saltin B (1971) Diet, muscle glycogen, and endurance performance. *Journal of Applied Physiology* 31:203–206.

Koopman R, Pannemans DLE, Jeukendrup AE, Gijsen AP, Senden JMG, Halliday D, Saris WHM, van Loon LJC, Wagenmakers AJM (2004) Combined ingestion of protein and carbohydrate improves protein balance during ultra-endurance exercise. *American Journal of Physiology, Endocrinology and Metabolism* 287:E712–720.

Lambert E, Speechley D, Dennis SC, Noakes T (1994) Enhanced endurance in trained cyclists during moderate intensity exercise following 2 weeks adaptation to a high fat diet. *European Journal of Applied Physiology* 69:287–293.

Miller W, Bryce R, Conlee R (1984) Adaptation to a high-fat diet that increases exercise endurance in male rats. *Journal of Applied Physiology* 56:78–83.

Muio D, Leddy J, Horvath P, Pendergast D (1994) Effect of dietary fat on metabolic adjustments to maximal VO2 and endurance in runners. *Medicine and Science in Sports and Exercise* 26:81–88.

Onywera V, Kiplamai F, Boit MK, Pitsiladis Y (2004) Food and macronutrient intake of elite distance runners. *International Journal of Sport Nutrition and Exercise Metabolism* 14(6):709–716.

Phinney S (2004) Ketogenic diets and physical performance. *Nutrition and Metabolism* 1:2. Electronic version online: www.nutritionandmetabolism.com/content/1/1/2, 2004.

Phinney S, Bistrian B, Evans W, Gervino E, Blackburn G (1983) The human metabolic response to chronic ketosis without caloric restriction: preservation of sub maximal exercise capability with reduced carbohydrate oxidation. *Metabolism* 32:769–776.

Robins A, Davies D, Jones G (2005) The effect of nutritional manipulation on ultra-endurance performance: a case study. *Research in Sports Medicine* 13(3):199–215.

Stubbs RJ, Hughes DA, Johnstone AM, Whybrow S, Horgan GW, King N, Blundell J (2004) Rate and extent of compensatory changes in energy intake and expenditure in response to altered exercise and diet composition in humans. *American Journal of Physiology: Regulatory and Integrated Comparative Physiology* 286(2):R350–358.

Xia G, Chin M, Girandola R, Liu R (2001) The effects of diet and supplements on a male world champion lightweight rower. *Journal of Sports Medicine and Physical Fitness* 41(2):223–228.

Zanker CL, Swaine IL (2000) Responses of bone turnover markers to repeated endurance running in humans under conditions of energy balance or energy restriction. *European Journal of Applied Physiology* 83:434–440.

CHAPTER THREE

Hormones

Some readers may be familiar with the *female athlete triad*, a complex that involves disordered eating, *amenorrhea* (loss of menses), and reduced bone mass. Far less common is awareness that male endurance athletes also are at risk for having reduced levels of reproductive hormones that may result in osteoporosis. Endurance athletes of both genders generally show reduced levels of reproductive hormones (estrogen and testosterone) in comparison to strength-power athletes or sedentary controls. Male gymnasts and weight lifters also have slightly lower testosterone levels than non-exercising subjects, but these levels return to baseline if training loads are reduced. Changes in hormone levels, then, appear to be the consequences of either the volume or type of exercise performed, not simply of exercise per se.

Estrogen and testosterone have multiple influences on bone, some of which are well understood while others remain undefined. In general, we know that both hormones reduce bone resorption and retard the overall rate at which bone remodeling occurs. This change in metabolic tempo is important, since the result of a remodeling cycle is net bone loss. Estrogen both reduces the number of formed osteoclasts (cells that break down bone) and decreases their lifespan. Reductions in estrogen levels lead to decreases in intestinal absorption and increased urinary excretion of calcium, both of which limit the availability of calcium for bone. Testosterone in males is converted to estrogen through a process known as *aromatization*. Although testosterone may have direct effects on bone, much of its skeletal influence could be indirect, through its action on muscle.

Testosterone

Testosterone is a steroid that is produced in both males and females. It plays a key role in physical and emotional health for both genders. On average, an adult male produces 40–60 times more testosterone than an adult female, but the female body is more sensitive to lower concentrations. From an athletic perspective, testosterone plays an important role in muscular strength development through its role in protein synthesis and in the production of red blood cells. Additionally, it is an important governor of body composition and improves recovery from exercise. Both men and women rely on testosterone to maintain libido, muscle mass, and bone density.

Testosterone secretion is initiated from the brain as the hypothalamus secretes gonadotropin-releasing hormone, which in turn stimulates the pituitary to secrete luteinizing hormone (LH). In men, LH acts on the testicles to induce the production of testosterone. Like other steroid hormones, testosterone is derived from cholesterol and is delivered to target tissues through the circulatory system, bound to sex hormone binding globulin (SHBG). Testosterone levels have a circadian rhythm in which values peak in the early morning. For this reason, if testing is required, every effort should be made to collect a blood sample at this time.

Short-duration, high-intensity interval training and resistance exercise cause acute increases in testosterone levels. Illustrating this point, Raastad and colleagues (2000) demonstrated that lifting with 3RM (Repetition Maximum, indicative of a high intensity workout) for squats and front squats, and at a rate of 6RM for leg extensions, induces a higher exercise-induced testosterone release than do the same exercises at 70% of resistance.

In contrast, prolonged physical or emotional stress, such as bicycle competitions lasting several days or sustained periods of military training, cause significant reductions in testosterone levels. For example, Opstad (1992) reported that plasma levels of testosterone and other androgenic hormones decreased by 60–80% during a five-day military operation with round-the-clock physical activity. These maneuvers produced a profound energy deficit, with the average daily energy expenditure estimated at 40,000 kJ (9,560 kcal), while intake was only 2,000 kJ (500 kcal).

Some studies of male endurance athletes demonstrate that testosterone levels are not suppressed chronically (Hetland, et al.,1993), while others indicate that long-term reduction in hormone levels does occur (Wheeler, 1984). For example, MacConnie and colleagues (1986) evaluated male marathon runners who were running

125–200 miles per week. They determined that hypothalamic gonadotropin releasing hormone (GnRH) levels were significantly decreased (GnRH is a neurohormone that influences the production of testosterone). These low levels were improved when mileage was reduced by 70%, but testosterone levels still remained low. A possible reason for these discrepancies in results is that testosterone levels and responses to a given exercise protocol depend on each athlete's training background. For example, adult hormone levels may be contingent on the time in which training was initiated (pre-pubertal versus post-pubertal), or be sensitive to the rate at which training volume or intensity is progressed. Reductions in testosterone levels have been reported in athletes running as little as 64 km per week.

In males, symptoms of low testosterone may include:

- Muscle loss/atrophy
- Fatigue
- Weight gain
- Memory loss
- Decreased libido
- Erectile dysfunction
- Frequent urination
- Dry skin

A simple blood test ordered by your physician can detect low testosterone levels.

Normal testosterone levels range from 298–1,098 ng/dl. Most physicians recommend treatment for low testosterone (hypogonadism) if levels are < 350 ng/dl. It is important to determine if hypogonadism is of the primary or secondary type. In primary hypogonadism, LH levels usually are elevated, indicating the problem is at the testicular level. In secondary hypogonadism, LH levels are low, indicating the problem lies in the brain.

Treatment options for endurance athletes with low testosterone levels may include relative rest, dietary modifications, and/or testosterone replacement. Commonly prescribed testosterone replacement formulations may be delivered by way of injections, skin patches, buccal (gum) absorption, or creams/gels.

Unfortunately, few long-term studies have evaluated the effectiveness of testosterone substitution therapy on the bone mass of males. The consensus at this time appears to be that, despite the normalization of circulating testosterone levels with replacement therapy, long-term bone mass still may be compromised in some individuals. This finding highlights the fact that bone mass is the result of multiple complex interactions and that testosterone is only one, albeit an important, consideration.

Historically, estrogen has been recognized as the key hormone governing bone cell activity in the female skeleton. It was assumed that testosterone played an equivalent role for males. However, in the mid-1990s, that view was challenged as selected cases of males with estrogen receptor and aromatase gene mutations were found to have incompletely developed skeletons and reduced bone mass. Bone mass improved in these males when they were provided supplemental estrogen. This information led researchers to consider that estrogen may be the more dominant hormone in the regulation of both the male and female skeleton. In the most recent studies of males it appears that estrogen is in fact the more important hormone regulating bone resorption, while both estrogen and testosterone are important for the modulation of bone formation through actions on the osteoblast.

Estrogen

Estrogen is the primary female reproductive hormone and occurs in the body in three forms: estradiol, estriol, and estrone. All three are produced by androgen precursors through the actions of specific enzymes. Estrogen is produced by the developing follicles in the ovaries following signals from follicle stimulating hormone (FSH) and luteinizing hormone (LH). The liver, adrenal glands, and adipose tissues also produce smaller quantities of some estrogens. Both genders synthesize estrogens, but they but are found in significantly higher concentrations in the menstruating female. Estrogen is considered a "pleiotropic" hormone, which means that is responsible for the regulation of multiple systems and capable of exerting effects on numerous body targets, including bone.

The recognition of severe bone loss in the female endurance athlete has been well studied and correlated with amenorrhea (absence of normal menstrual cycle) and therefore reduced estrogen levels. Females who start training before menarche, train the most intensively, consume few calories, and have low body masses (Snow-Harter, 1994) are at higher risk for amenorrhea. Individuals who participate in sports that emphasize aesthetics or low body weight, such as figure skating, distance running, or cycling, are at greatest risk. Although many alternative mechanisms have been proposed to explain why female athletes lose their menstrual cycle and thus the protective effect of estrogen on bone mass, the energy-deficit theory appears most plausible. Among studies reporting such outcomes, Cobb and colleagues (2003) found that osteopenia occurred in 48% of female runners who had menstrual irregularity compared with 26% of women who had regular menstrual cycles.

Clinical studies that control strictly for energy intakes and expenditures reveal that negative energy balance is the primary underlying cause of menstrual irregularities. Researchers have determined that 30 kcal per kilogram of lean body mass is the threshold below which hormonal perturbations are known to occur. It is important to understand that an energy deficit may be created either by inadequate dietary intake (dieting, anorexia, disordered eating) or through exercise expenditure, or a combination of both.

Symptoms of energy deficit and thus reduced levels of reproductive hormones are those typically described in the overtraining literature and include:

- Illness/injury
- Lack of interest in training
- Failure to improve
- Sluggishness/heavy legs
- Irritability/depression
- Increased hunger/thirst
- Decreased libido
- Decreased exercise heart rate

Despite the correlation between amenorrhea and low bone mass, some studies have found that low bone mass may be present in female athletes with normal menstrual cycles. That is, bone mineral status may be diminished prior to any overt signs of menstrual cycle disturbance. More specifically and seriously, regularly menstruating female athletes with high levels of dietary restraint show lower levels of BMD (bone mineral density) than those with normal eating behaviors (Cobb, et al., 2003). A survey conducted by Kiernan and colleagues (1992) on 2,459 male and 1,786 female American runners showed that 8% of males and 24% of females had increased scores on a questionnaire designed to detect abnormal eating attitudes. The mechanisms by which an energy deficit leads to reductions in bone mass now have been defined. Based on markers of bone cell activity, both reductions in bone formation and increases in bone resorption increase as the degree of energy deficit is increased (Ihle and Loucks, 2004).

Many female endurance athletes are recommended to take prescription oral contraceptives in attempt to improve low levels of estrogen and thus spare bone (Liu and Lebrun, 2006). Despite variable improvement (1–19%) in bone mineral density with hormonal intervention, a complete review of 26 published studies revealed that no treatment resulted in restoration of bone mass to that of age-matched controls (Vescovi and De Souza, 2008). Review of the scientific literature shows that "the most successful and indeed essential strategy for improving BMD in women with functional amenorrhea is to increase caloric intake such that body mass is increased and there is a resumption of menses." As our former colleague, Dr. Margot Putukian, MD, now Director of Athletic Medicine at Princeton University says, "You need to make food your friend."

Summary

Both male and female endurance athletes are at risk for reduced levels of reproductive hormones that are known to influence bone mass and strength favorably. The submaximal and prolonged nature of endurance exercise appears to reduce reproductive hormone levels as compared to short duration, high intensity modes of exercise. The physical and emotional stress related to acute or prolonged energy deficit may lead to rapid and irreversible reductions in reproductive hormone levels for both genders. Improvements in reproductive hormone levels may be realized through dietary and training program modifications. Restoration of energy balance in both genders and resumption of menses in females appears imperative for re-establishment of bone cell activity and skeletal health. Supplemental hormone replacement may be warranted in certain cases, but scientific studies do not support this intervention as being completely effective in improving bone parameters.

REFERENCES

Cobb KL, Bachrach LK, Greendale G, Marcus R, Neer RM, Nieves J, Sowers MF, Brown BW, Gopalkrishnan G, Luetters L, Tanner HK, Ward B, Kelsey JR (2003) Disordered eating, menstrual irregularity, and bone mineral density in female runners. *Medicine and Science in Sport and Exercise* 35:711–719.

Hackney A (1998) Testosterone and reproductive dysfunction in endurance-trained men. In: *Encyclopedia of Sports Medicine and Science*, TD Fahey (editor). Internet Society for Sport Science, September 20, sportssci.org.

Hetland ML, Haarbo J, Christiansen C (1993) Low bone mass and high bone turnover in male long distance runners. *Journal of Clinical Endocrinology and Metabolism* 77:770–775.

Ihle R, Loucks AB (2004) Dose-response relationships between energy availability and bone turnover in young exercising women. *Journal of Bone and Mineral Research* 19:1231–1240.

Kiernan M, Rodin J, Brownell KD, Wilmore JH, Crandall C (1992) Relation of level of exercise, age, and weight-cycling history to weight and eating concerns in male and female runners. *Health Psychology* 11:418–421.

Liu S, Lebrun C (2006) Effect of oral contraceptives and hormone replacement therapy on bone mineral density in premenopausal and perimenopausal women: a systemic review. *British Journal of Sports Medicine* 40:11–24. 200

MacConnie SE, Barkan A, Lampman RM, Schork MA, Beitins IZ (1986) Decreased hypothalamic gonadotropin-releasing hormone secretion in male marathon runners. *New England Journal of Medicine* 315:411–417.

Opstad PK (1992) Androgenic hormones during prolonged physical stress, sleep, and energy deficiency. *Journal of Clinical Endocrinology and Metabolism* 74(5):1176–1183.

Raastad T, Bjoro T, Hallen J (2000) Hormonal responses to high and moderate intensity strength exercise. *European Journal of Applied Physiology* 82(1–2):121–128.

Seeman E, Szmukler G, Formica C, Tsalamandris C, Mestrovic R (1992) Osteoporosis in anorexia nervosa: the influence of peak bone density, bone loss, oral contraceptive use, and exercise. *Journal of Bone and Mineral Research* 7:1467–1474.

Snow-Harter CM (1994) Bone health and prevention of osteoporosis in active and athletic women. *Clinical Sports Medicine* 13:389–404.

Vescovi J, De Souza M (2008) Strategies to reverse bone loss in women with functional hypothalamic amenorrhea: a systematic review of the literature. *Osteoporosis International* 19(4):465–478.

Wheeler GD, Wall SR, Belcastro AN, Cumming DC (1994) Reduced serum testosterone and prolactin levels in male distance runners. *Journal of the American Medical Association* 252:514–516.

CHAPTER FOUR

Energy Balance and Metabolism

The single greatest factor in the development of osteoporosis in the endurance athlete is probably chronic energy deficit. It is critical for athletes to strive to achieve energy balance and to understand its relationship to diet and exercise expenditure. The key process at work in this relationship is metabolism.

Metabolism comprises the living body's cellular processes and chemical reactions, and heat is its end product. Thus, metabolic rate is expressed in terms of the amount of heat liberated from the sum of these reactions during a standardized period of time. The food we eat has the potential to be either stored or used as energy after being converted to ATP. However, the metabolism of our food into ATP requires energy, and a side effect of this conversion is release of heat. Additional heat-producing reactions that occur during exercise include muscle contraction, blood circulation, sweating, and maintenance of pH. Essentially all body processes that use energy also liberate heat.

The unit *calorie* is used to quantify the energy released from foods or expended during exercise. A calorie (small "c") is the quantity of heat required to raise the temperature of 1 g of water by 1°C. Because this is such a small unit, the *kilocalorie* (kcal or capital C), equal to 1,000 calories, is a more useful unit for describing energy metabolism.

An athlete's metabolic rate can be determined by measuring the quantity of heat that is liberated over a given period of time. In research institutions this is accomplished in a specially constructed chamber known as a direct *calorimeter*. Because direct calorimetry is expensive and rarely available to the general public, most athletes use a more practical method of measuring body metabolism.

Because most physiologic processes involve reactions of food with oxygen, total body metabolic rate can be calculated from the rate at which oxygen is utilized.

Metabolizing enough glucose, fat, or protein to combine with 1l of oxygen releases 4.825 Calories. This quantity is known as the *energy equivalent* of oxygen. Using this energy equivalent, heat liberation by the body can be determined indirectly by measuring the amount of oxygen utilized.

An athlete's total energy expenditure equals the sum of *basal metabolic rate* (BMR) plus energy used in daily living activities, food metabolism, and exercise. BMR refers to the amount of energy required to maintain physiologic processes of the body while at rest. To determine BMR, oxygen utilization is measured over a period of time when a person is awake but lying still and free of emotional distraction. Although variable and dependent on body size (lean body mass) an average BMR is in the range of 1,400–1,800 kcal. The amount of energy expended with activities of daily living can be quite variable and depends on one's employment and leisure pursuits. After a meal is consumed, metabolic rate increases as a result of the chemical reactions associated with digestion, absorption, and storage of food. This is known as the *thermic effect of food*. Metabolism increases by about 10% following a meal.

A standard formula for estimating resting energy expenditure is body weight in pounds multiplied by 11 (or kilograms multiplied by 22). For simplicity, we will consider *resting energy expenditure* (REE) as the sum of all metabolic expenditure excluding purposeful exercise, or approximately:

115 lb X 11 = 1,265 kcal

125 lb X 11 = 1,375 kcal

135 lb X 11 = 1,485 kcal

145 lb X 11 = 1,595 kcal

155 lb X 11 = 1,705 kcal

165 lb X 11 = 1,815 kcal

175 lb X 11 = 1,925 kcal

185 lb X 11 = 2,035 kcal

195 lb X 11 = 2,145 kcal

205 lb X 11 = 2,255 kcal

215 lb X 11 = 2,365 kcal

225 lb X 11 = 2,475 kcal

An athlete can determine exercise energy expenditure with reasonable accuracy by using a heart rate monitor. We have had experience with the Polar heart rate monitor (Polar Electro Inc., www.polarusa.com). Using this device, an athlete enters data for gender, weight, height, and activity level into a wrist computer. The device calculates and displays caloric expenditure based on an internal mathematical algorithm and exercising heart rate. Keytel and colleagues (2005) concluded that it is also possible to estimate physical activity energy expenditure "with a great deal of accuracy" by monitoring heart rate, provided that adjustments for age, gender, body mass, and fitness are made.

A case study will help athletes appreciate the needs of their bodies for food energy to offset exercise expenditure. Consider a 24-year-old female weighing 125 pounds who is a category II cyclist with an REE of 1,374 kcal. She follows this weekly exercise routine:

Saturday: 40 mile road race, 112 minutes (HR 162), expenditure = 2,015 kcal

Sunday: 45 minute recovery ride (HR 120), expenditure = 626 kcal

Monday: 180 minute ride (HR 142), expenditure = 2,854 kcal

Tuesday: 120 minute ride (HR 132), 6 X 2" intervals (HR 178), expenditure = 2,812 kcal

Wednesday: 45 minute recovery ride (HR 118), expenditure = 626 kcal

Thursday: Day off

Friday: 25 mile time trial, 64 minutes (HR 169), expenditure = 1,253 kcal

Her total energy expenditure (REE + exercise expenditure) is:

Saturday: 3,390 kcal

Sunday: 2,001 kcal

Monday: 4,229 kcal

Tuesday: 4,187 kcal

Wednesday: 2,001 kcal

Thursday: 1,375 kcal

Friday: 2,682 kcal

Table 4.1 shows two sample diets that approximately meet the energy requirements for Monday, when total energy expenditure was

Table 4.1 Sample diets for monday

	High Carbohydrate	Moderate Carbohydrate
Breakfast	2 eggs 2 c oatmeal 1 banana 2 c skim milk	2 eggs with 2 tsp olive oil 1 c oatmeal 1 banana 1 c skim milk 3 tbsp walnuts
Snack	2 c Greek yogurt 2 c red potatoes 2 c strawberries 2 tbsp walnuts	1 c Greek yogurt 1 c red potatoes 2 c strawberries ½ c walnuts
Lunch	12" turkey club sandwich with vegetables (lettuce and tomato) and black olives 2 c mixed berries 2 tbsp walnuts	6" turkey club sandwich with vegetables (lettuce and tomato) and black olives; ¼ c sunflower seeds
Snack	2 oz corn chips with ¾ c black bean salsa 2 c skim milk 1 ½ oz shredded cheese 2 c red grapes	1 oz corn chips with ½ c black bean salsa 2 c skim milk 1 c red grapes ½ avocado
Dinner	5 oz salmon 2 c brown rice 2 c mixed salad greens 2 oranges	5 oz salmon 1 c brown rice 1 c mixed salad greens with 1 tbsp olive oil 2 oranges
Snack	2 c Greek yogurt 1 yam 2 apples 1 tbsp flax seed	1 c Greek yogurt 1 yam 1 apple with 2 tbsp nut butter 10–12 macadamia nuts

equal to 4,229 kcal. Both high carbohydrate and moderate carbohydrate examples are included.

This case study shows that an athlete may easily require twice the resting daily requirement. During the 2008 Beijing Olympics, Michael Phelps stated in a television interview that his target caloric intake was 10,000–12,000 kcal per day. Tour de France riders' energy requirements have been estimated in the 7,000 kcal per day range. In truth, precise energy balance on a daily basis may be difficult for athletes to achieve, but purposeful attempts must be made in order to maintain long-term equilibrium.

We stress that bone health is contingent upon energy balance, and if exercise expenditure exceeds dietary intake, bone loss results. Again, the single greatest factor in the development of osteoporosis in the endurance athlete is probably chronic energy deficit. In 2006, researchers from Japan (Montanaga and colleagues) utilized the heart rate monitor method of estimating energy expenditure in a group of male middle and long-distance runners. Their mean total energy expenditure (TEE) was 4,514 +/− 739 kcal/day and energy intake (EI) was only 3,784 +/− 91 kcal/day, resulting in an energy deficit (expenditure is greater than intake) of over 700 kcal/day. These objective findings support the observations of other researchers that most endurance athletes exist in a 15–25% energy deficit state. Nutrition and bone expert Dr. Anne Loucks (2007, p. 348) from Ohio University has had this to say about energy deficit:

> Many marathon runners and other endurance athletes reduce energy availability either (i) intentionally to modify body size and composition for improving performance; (ii) compulsively in a psychopathological pattern of disordered eating; or (iii) inadvertently because there is no strong biological drive to match energy intake to activity-induced energy expenditure. Inadvertent low energy availability is more extreme when consuming a low fat, high carbohydrate diet.

Failure to provide essential dietary energy may result in some or all of the following:

- Delayed recovery from training
- Stagnation in performance
- Signs and symptoms consistent with overtraining
- Increased incidence of "overuse injury"
- Slow recovery from injuries
- Reduced levels of reproductive hormones
- Increased incidence of menstrual cycle disturbance
- Loss of lean body mass
- Reductions in bone formation
- Increased rates of bone resorption
- Increased incidence of stress fractures
- Accelerated loss of bone mass/osteoporosis

Summary

It is important for endurance athletes to understand the importance of energy balance as it relates to dietary intake and exercise expenditure. In order to determine overall energy availability, compare your dietary intake with your exercise expenditure using the following steps:

1. To calculate your daily caloric intake, maintain a food log by recording all the food and energy-containing beverages you consume for one to three days.
2. Determine caloric and nutritional intake manually or with commercially available computer software.
3. Calculate exercise energy expenditure with a heart rate monitor.
4. Calculate the difference between intake and expenditure. The result is your overall energy availability.

You should consider the accumulation of frequent daily deficits or a chronic deficit a significant risk factor for bone loss as well as for suboptimal recovery or performance. Monitoring body composition with a bioelectrical impedance scale or skin fold assessment may provide further information about an athlete's energy status.

REFERENCES

Fogelholm M, Sievanen H, Heinonen A, Virtanen M, Uusi-Rasi K, Pasanen M, Vuori I (1997) Association between weight cycling history and bone mineral density in premenopausal women. *Osteoporosis International* 7(4):354–358.

Grinspoon S, Baum H, Kim V, Coggins C, Klibanski A (1995) Decreased bone formation and increased mineral dissolution during acute fasting in young women. *Journal of Clinical Endocrinology and Metabolism* 80:3628–3633.

Keytel L, Goedecke J, Noakes T, Hiiloskorpi H, Laukkanen R, van der Merwe L, Lambert E (2005) Prediction of energy expenditure from heart rate monitoring during submaximal exercise. *Journal of Sports Science* 23(3):289–297.

Laughlin G, Yen S (1996) Nutritional and endocrine-metabolic aberrations in amenorrheic athletes. *Journal of Clinical Endocrinology and Metabolism* 81:4301–4309.

Loucks A (2007) Low energy availability in the marathon and other endurance sports. *Sports Medicine* 37(4–5):348–352.

Montanaga K, Yoshida S, Yamagami F, Kawano T, Takeda E (2006) Estimation of total daily energy expenditure and its components by monitoring the heart rate of Japanese endurance athletes. *Journal of Nutritional Science and Vitaminology* 52(5):360–367.

Pritchard J, Nowson C, Wark J (1996) Bone loss accompanying diet-induced or exercise-induced weight loss: a randomized controlled study. *International Journal of Obesity Related Metabolic Disorders* 20(6):513–520.

Schlemmer A, Hassager C (1999) Acute fasting diminishes the circadian rhythm of biochemical markers of bone resorption. *European Journal of Endocrinology* 140:332–337.

Zanker C, Swaine I (1998) Relation between bone turnover, oestradiol, and energy balance in women distance runners. *British Journal of Sports Medicine* 32:167–171.

CHAPTER FIVE

Protein

The word protein is derived from the Greek word meaning "of prime importance" and this distinction may be accurate in the case of an endurance athlete's skeleton. Structurally, protein is composed of 21 particular amino acid building blocks. Some of these, the *essential amino acids*, must be consumed through the diet, while others can be manufactured by the body and thus are considered *nonessential*. Skeletal muscle represents 60–70% of the body's total protein stores, but nearly all tissues, including hormones and the collagen matrix of bone, are composed mainly of proteins.

The average sedentary adult is advised to consume 0.4–0.5 g of protein per pound of body weight per day, while most sports nutritionists believe that athletes require slightly more and recommend intakes in the 0.6–0.7 g/pound per day range (1.3–1.5 g/kg). It commonly is believed that "a typical diet" achieves this level of intake and supports both health and performance. Nonetheless, examination of the diet histories of many endurance athletes, including the elite, reveals that protein intake often falls at or below these levels. As one example of threshold protein intake, Onywera and colleagues (2005) reported the protein intake for an elite group of Kenyan distance runners at 1.3 g/kg of body mass per day. Their protein consumption represented approximately 10% of their overall daily energy intake.

In the past, serious concerns have been raised regarding "excessive" protein intake, since increases in dietary protein have been correlated with elevated rates of both bone cell remodeling and calcium excretion. This outcome was attributed to the reductions in body pH, *metabolic acidosis*, which results from the digestion of proteins containing certain amino acids. Notably, however, these findings were the outcome of tests performed in laboratory settings where subjects were fed purified protein supplements rather than whole foods. In contrast, studies investigating the diets of people eating real food, not synthetic laboratory food, reveal no bone loss despite higher than recommended protein intakes. In fact, most large-scale epidemiological and cross-sectional studies show that higher levels of protein intake promote increased bone mass and overall skeletal health. Although the exact mechanisms have yet to be fully defined, the results of Ammann and colleagues (2000) show that dietary protein influences growth factors including IGF-1 (Insulin growth factor-1) that are known to be highly anabolic to bone.

In 2000, Kerstetter and colleagues evaluated the effects on calcium status of graded protein intakes of 0.7, 0.8, 0.9, and 1.0 g/kg. They found that the former recommendation of .8 g/kg (0.4–0.5 g/lb) resulted in negative calcium homeostasis and suggested 0.9 g/kg was the lowest level at which a favorable calcium balance was observed. This study was conducted on eight healthy females who were allowed to eat whole foods. Protein intake was divided between animal and vegetable sources and calcium levels were controlled. The study subjects were not athletes, nor did they exercise during the study. Although such studies provide guidelines for the lower limits of protein necessary for bone health, there are few studies that define the safe upper or optimal protein requirement for athletes or those interested in increasing bone mass. The traditional recommended protein intake even for sedentary individuals probably is lower than ideal for the maintenance of bone health.

Scientists believe that protein balance exists when protein intake is equal to protein excretion. In a state of positive protein balance, intake exceeds excretion, with the additional protein available for the repair and synthesis of tissues including muscle and bone. Prolonged or intense endurance exercise stimulates whole body protein turnover (synthesis and degradation) and increases the oxidation of certain amino acids known collectively as the *branched chain amino acids* (BCAA). Protein turnover during exercise is affected by training status as well as an athlete's nutritional state. Well-trained athletes demonstrate less protein turnover during exercise than do those who are not trained. Supplemental carbohydrate consumed during exercise blunts protein turnover during exercise. More recently, studies have determined that habitual protein intake also decreases protein turnover during and following exercise.

In 2005 Bolster and colleagues conducted a landmark study by evaluating how habitual dietary protein intake influences skeletal muscle turnover following endurance exercise in five trained males. Each of the athletes followed three different diets, with varying amounts of protein, for four weeks time. Low protein (LP = 0.8g/kg), moderate protein (MP = 1.8g/kg), and high protein (HP = 3.6g/kg) diets were equal in total calories; only the macronutrient distribution was varied. Substrate oxidation was determined after three weeks on each of the diets. The synthesis rate of muscle was measured after a 75-minute endurance run performed at 70% VO2. Fractional synthetic rate (a measure of protein turnover) was significantly greater for LP (0.083%/hr) and MP (0.078%/hr) than for HP (0.052%/hr). This research supports the idea that protein intake plays a direct role in regulating skeletal muscle protein metabolism, while suggesting that moderately higher levels of protein intake may exert some sort of protective effect by reducing turnover.

In a similar but more recent study conducted by the U.S. Army (Pikosky, et al., 2008) male volunteers were provided diets containing either 0.9g/kg or 1.8g/kg of protein per day for 11 days. After four days to adapt to each of the diet conditions, the subjects were exposed to an exercise-induced energy deficit of 1,000 kcal for seven consecutive days. Exercise intensity was 50–65% VO2 max. Protein balance was measured, with the results demonstrating that protein balance was maintained in the 1.8 g/kg group but negative in the 0.9 g/kg group.

These studies indicate that habitual protein consumption above the level traditionally recommended can reduce the catabolic state that is induced with endurance exercise. However, as we have discussed, protein intake and skeletal health are modulated by a variety of factors including the overall dietary pH and the amount of calcium consumed in the diet. Table 5.1 provides a list of studies that have evaluated different levels of protein consumption in strength and endurance exercise.

The research on both humans and animals documents that it is reasonable and safe for endurance athletes to consume dietary protein at levels of approximately 0.9–1.2 g per pound of body weight (or 1.8–2.4 g/kg). This requirement may need to be slightly modified in times of increased or decreased training loads. We recommend that if you are new to exercise and/or if you are a well-conditioned athlete undergoing an increase in training volume, you should consider targeting the upper end of the protein requirement. The lower level of the recommended range might be adequate for times of reduced training or after fully adapting to an increased training load. Table 5.2 lists excellent food sources of protein.

To calculate your individual daily protein requirement, multiply your body weight in pounds by 0.9–1.2 or in kilograms by 1.8–2.4. For example, for a 150-pound athlete: 150 X 0.9–1.2 = 135–180 g/day. To consume protein in this range, this athlete could consume daily:

- 2 eggs (12 g)
- 2 cups skim milk (16 g)
- 6 oz Tofu (18 g)
- 1 chicken breast (30 g)
- 6 oz tuna (44 g)
- 4 oz lean beef (24 g)

Table 5.1 Summary of studies evaluating protein levels in athletes

Author(s)	Protein levels	Findings
Fern	1.3, 3.3 g/kg	3.3 g/kg produced greater muscle gains.
Tarnopolsky, et al.	0.9, 1.4, 2.4 g/kg	1.4 g/kg produced better muscle gains than 0.9 g/kg. No additional increase with 2.4 g/kg.
Bigard, et al.	1.5, 2.5 g/kg	Serum amino acid decline is prevented post-exercise with 2.5 g/kg.
Bolster, et al.	0.8, 1.8, 3.6 g/kg	Less protein was oxidized following exercise in athletes consuming 3.6 than 0.8 g/kg.
Pikosky, et al.	0.9, 1.8 g/kg	Protein balance was maintained with 1.8 but negative with 0.9 g/kg.

Note: The references at the end of this chapter give full publication data.

Table 5.2 Protein-rich food sources

Protein-rich food source	Serving size	Protein (g)
Tuna	3 oz	22
Lean beef	3 oz	18
Whole egg	1 large	6
Yogurt	1 cup	11
Tofu	4 oz	15
Peanut butter	1 tbsp	4
Lentils	½ cup	9

Several years ago we noticed an up-and-coming female ultra-runner named Francesca Conte who was featured in Neal Jamison's book, *Running Through The Wall* (Breakaway Books, 2003). At that time, Dr. Conte had been running ultras for two years but had experienced early success, including a fifth place overall finish and win in the female division at the Arkansas 100-mile race. In Jamison's book she detailed the importance of her diet, which she described as being "high-protein Mediterranean style." Over the years Dr. Conte has continued to accumulate an impressive number of ultrarunning accomplishments, including a 2008 win at the USATF 50-mile national championships.

Recently, Dr. Conte was very generous in explaining to us some of the details of her training diet. To date, Dr. Conte has completed over 40 ultras, including multiple hundred milers; she averages five races per year and trains by running between 60–115 miles per week. She attempts to consume at least 100 g of protein per day when engaged in higher volume training. Typical protein sources for her include chicken, fish (raw or cooked), red meat (once every two to three weeks), and vegetarian sources including hummus. When asked about her dairy and soy intake she said yes to both in approximately a 70:30 ratio. Her soy consumption includes chocolate soy milk (Silk) and occasionally tofu. She drinks whole dairy milk; she says, "I would rather hit myself with a hammer than drink skim milk." Additionally, she utilizes a protein drink that she purchases at a local health food store that contains "as few ingredients as possible (i.e., 'natural')." To complement her protein intake, she includes pasta with tomato sauce, potatoes, large salads, fruit, and olive oil.

When asked if there was any additional advice she would like to include, she relayed that the way she grew up eating taught her what and when, and that philosophy has helped her performance. Additionally, she is a firm believer that food should be real and as local as possible and that, ultimately, anyone who eats real food for more than a few weeks will know the difference between what they should and should not eat. Dr. Conte earned a PhD in Biology from the University of Virgnia and, along with her partner and professional ultrarunner Gil, owns Bad to the Bone Endurance Sports and the Charlottesville Running Company (francesca@charlottesvillerunningcompany.com).

In addition to the overall quantity of dietary protein consumed, there are other qualitative considerations with respect to the protein choices that are related to endurance performance and bone health. Protein "quality" can be described in a variety of ways, each of which has both advantages and disadvantages. A protein's *biologic value* is defined by the proportion of absorbed protein from a food source that is utilized for maintenance and growth. The biologic value of protein in a food is variable and depends on multiple factors, including the presence of other nutrients (vitamins and minerals) or the quantity of the protein's various amino acids.

Vitamins and minerals are critical for the synthesis of new tissues, so dietary deficiencies can severely reduce a protein's biologic value. In a similar way, if specific amino acids in food are limited, the synthesis (or repair) of body tissues from a particular protein is limited to this degree. This is known as a *rate-limiting* amino acid. As such, amino acids that are available above the level of the rate-limiting amino acid are of no biologic value other than as a source of calories. Lastly, the nutritional status and particular metabolism of an individual influence a protein's inherent biologic value. Age, health, gender, body mass, training status, and hormonal levels may all influence how fully any particular individual can utilize a protein. The biologic values for some excellent protein sources are:

- Whey protein: 100
- Soy bean: 96
- Chicken egg: 94
- Cow milk: 90
- Rice: 83
- Fish: 76
- Beef: 74
- Casein: 71
- Tofu (soy curd): 64

Essential Amino Acids

Essential amino acids cannot be synthesized in the body and therefore must be consumed in the diet. Isoleucine, leucine, and valine are three notable essential amino acids known as the branched chain amino acids (BCAAs). They serve as precursors for the synthesis of glutamine and alanine, two other amino acids that are used in large quantities during prolonged or intense exercise. The essential amino acids are:

- Histidine
- Isoleucine*
- Leucine*
- Lysine

- Methionine
- Phenylalanine
- Threonine
- Tryptophan
- Valine*

    *Branched chain amino acid

In a study conducted by Coombes and McNaughton (2000), two groups of research subjects performed two hours of stationary bike riding. The experimental group had taken a daily BCAA supplement for the preceding 14 days while the control group was provided with a placebo. Both groups demonstrated significant increases in biomarkers of muscle damage lasting up to five days. However, the extent of the muscle damage was significantly lower in the BCAA supplemental group. Subsequently, in 2008 Negro and colleagues suggested that because BCAAs decrease exercise-induced muscle damage, promote muscle protein synthesis, reduce delayed onset muscle soreness, and alter immune system responses, they should be considered useful supplements for athletes.

Glutamine is the most abundant amino acid in blood and comprises more than 60% of the free amino acid pool in muscle tissue. It is classified as a non-essential amino acid because it can be synthesized by the body at various sites, including in skeletal muscle, the liver, and the brain. However, some authorities consider it to be a "conditionally essential" amino acid because synthesis by the body may be inadequate in certain circumstances.

The stress of exercise is known to increase dramatically the body's need for glutamine. The fact that glutamine is an important nutrient for the immune system is also now well documented. Glutamine levels are significantly reduced following prolonged exercise and in athletes who train intensively glutamine levels may be chronically low. Some studies have linked deficiencies in glutamine with poor performance and diminished immunity. The best sources of glutamine from whole foods include lean sources of animal protein, dairy products, beans, legumes, and some vegetables, including raw cabbage, spinach, and beets (see Table 5.3).

Whey Protein

Whey protein is the collection of globular proteins that can be isolated from whey, a by-product of the manufacture of cheese from

Table 5.3 Glutamine content in select foods

Food	Portion	Glutamine (g)
Lean beef	3 oz	4.05
Chicken breast	3 oz	3.74
Skim milk	1 cup	1.67
Lentils	½ cup	1.39
Soy milk	1 cup	1.35
Whole egg	1 large	0.82

cow's milk. Whey protein is available in three major forms: concentrate, isolate, and hydrolysate. Concentrates contain low levels of fat, cholesterol, and carbohydrate (lactose). They are the least expensive of the whey options and range in protein content from 30% to 80% by weight. Isolates are 90% protein by weight because they have been further processed to remove fat and carbohydrate. Hydrolysates are partially hydrolyzed (broken down by combination with water) and predigested, and as a result can be absorbed at a faster rate.

Because of its high biologic value and rapid rate of absorption, whey protein has gained increased popularity in the medical community and sports nutrition supplement industry. Reportedly, whey protein is being used in treatment of cancer, HIV, hepatitis B, cardiovascular disease, and osteoporosis. Also reported as a result of whey protein consumption are improvements in body composition, reductions in muscle damage, and improvements in immune system function following exercise. Scientists believe that the primary mechanism by which whey exerts its effects is the intracellular conversion of the amino acid cysteine to glutathione, a powerful intracellular antioxidant. Relevant experimental studies in this area include work by Middleton and colleagues (2004). They evaluated the role of whey protein isolate on glutathione concentrations in whole blood as well as in peripheral mononuclear cell populations during six weeks of aerobic training in 18 male cyclists. The training stress resulted in significantly lower glutathione concentrations in whole blood, but this effect was mitigated with whey supplementation. Whey supplementation also produced a significant increase in mononuclear cell glutathione following a simulated cycling time trial of 40 km.

Because whey protein is easily dissolved in fluids, it often is incorporated into supplemental drinks to be used during or immediately following exercise. Some research suggests that the use of a small amount of protein in conjunction with supplemental carbohydrate during exercise improves endurance performance and reduces subsequent muscle damage. However, research on the use of protein during exercise is inconsistent and there have been numerous studies reporting that protein affords no benefit above the use of carbohydrate alone.

When the scientific community has produced no clear consensus on a particular subject we like to consult the real experts—endurance athletes with practical experience. In conversations with a number of endurance and ultra-endurance athletes we believe there is some general agreement on the issue of protein consumption during training and competition. Most athletes do not feel that there is significant value in using supplemental protein during events lasting less than four hours. This is especially true for events involving running (marathon, international distance triathlon), since protein may increase the likelihood of gastrointestinal disturbance.

For events lasting between four and 12 hours, including ultramarathon running, half- and full-length ironman distance triathlon, ultra cycling/rowing, and adventure racing, environmental conditions often dictate whether protein is utilized. As temperature and humidity increase, most athletes lean toward less protein because physiologic stress is high and digestion/absorption is more difficult. When environmental conditions are less extreme, many endurance athletes feel that their rate of recovery will be enhanced if they incorporate some protein into their fueling routine. Most athletes participating in events lasting longer than 12 hours (ultra distance events), including multiple day events such as the bike race across America or a multiple day triathlon (ultraman), consider protein supplementation absolutely mandatory to minimize lean tissue catabolism and maintain performance.

Despite the consensus of athletes themselves regarding the use of supplemental protein during exercise, some advocates of this strategy are hesitant about the use of dairy-based whey. For example, *The Endurance Athlete's Guide to Success* offers the following statements about protein use during exercise:

> We recommend a combination of both soy and whey protein, used at separate times, to provide the most comprehensive support for an endurance athlete's diet. We believe that whey protein is the premier for recovery and enhanced immune system function, while soy protein is ideal for fulfilling protein requirements prior

to and during endurance exercise. Because it (soy) has less potential than whey protein for producing ammonia, a primary cause
of muscle fatigue, soy protein is best used prior to and during exercise. Although not as high in concentration as whey protein,
soy protein still provides a substantial amount of branched chain
amino acids, which your body readily converts for energy production. Soy protein also has a high level of aspartic acid, which plays
an important role in energy production via the Krebs cycle. Lastly,
soy protein has higher levels of phenylalanine than does whey,
which may aid in maintaining alertness during extreme ultra distance races. (99)

The mechanism by which whey protein influences bone mass
has not been well defined. Most of the studies evaluating whey-
bone interaction have used animal subjects rather than humans
and have been relatively short term. It remains unclear whether
whey protein influences the overall rate of bone remodeling activity or acts specifically on osteoblasts or osteoclasts. Whey protein may affect bone indirectly through improvements in skeletal
muscle strength.

Soy Protein

Whole soy foods have received considerable attention for their
role in disease prevention, especially in relation to heart disease
and osteoporosis. Soybeans contain isoflavones, a subclass of flavonoids, which have a chemical structure similar to the hormone
estrogen. Isoflavones are rare in nature and exist in nutritionally
relevant amounts only in soybeans. The primary isoflavones in soy
are genistein, daidzein, and glycitein. A serving of soy food (tofu,
tempeh) contains approximately 30 mg of isoflavones whereas isolated soy protein contains approximately 2 mg isoflavone/gram of
protein. Isoflavones may bind to estrogen receptor sites in the body
and influence estrogen-regulated gene products. As a result they
are often called plant estrogens (*phytoestrogens*). Bone cells are
known to possess estrogen receptor sites. Research appears to confirm that soy's influence on bone is mediated through isoflavone
pathways.

Human feeding studies suggest that, based on urinary markers,
soy inhibits bone turnover and/or increases bone formation rates
as well as increases bone mineral density in perimenopausal or
postmenopausal females. The majority of the benefit appears to be
limited to the spine.

In addition to the isoflavone-mediated pathways, soy protein digestion does not induce the reductions in body pH that are typical of animal or dairy-based protein sources. As we have discussed, the digestion of certain proteins incorporating sulfur-containing amino acids (methionine and cysteine) may have the potential to induce a metabolic acidosis, which results in an increase in calcium excretion. The fact that soy protein is relatively low in these sulfur-containing amino acids may explain why this particular protein source is especially beneficial for bone (Bawa, 2010). These findings reinforce the earlier research of Breslau and colleagues (1988), who fed human subjects, in random, order three different diets containing similar amounts of protein and calcium over 12 days. They found that subjects excreted 150, 121, and 103 mg of calcium over 24 hours when on the animal protein, mixed, and soy protein diets respectively.

Despite the protective role soy protein appears to play in cardiovascular and bone health, some experts oppose its consumption for fear of its estrogenizing effects. Although phytoestrogens from soy are chemically similar to estrogen, they do not initiate the same biological effects as endogenous estrogen. Paradoxically, phytoestrogens act as anti-estrogens in the body, as they may limit binding sites that would normally be occupied by true estrogen hormones. The general recommendation for females with elevated risk of estrogen-dependent cancer is to consume limited quantities of whole soy foods and to avoid supplemental soy isoflavones. There appears to be no scientific merit to support the contention that soy protein reduces male testosterone levels (Messina, 2010).

Diets that are high in acid-producing foods, including many sources of protein, can cause excessive urinary calcium loss related to metabolic acidosis. Calcium loss is directly related to urinary net acid excretion. Although increased dietary protein will likely create an obligatory calcium loss, this may be offset by a number of factors (dietary pH, phosphate), including an appropriate level of calcium in the diet. In a presentation at the annual meeting of the American Society for Bone and Mineral Research in September, 1997, recognized bone researcher Linda Massey (2008) recommended a dietary calcium-to-protein ratio of more than 20:1 (mg:g). She recommended that, for a 150-pound athlete with a protein requirement of 135 g per day, daily calcium intake should be 2,700 mg (135 x 20 = 2,700 mg). Table 5.4 shows the calcium content protein-rich foods. As you can see, in order to maintain the suggested ratio of 20:1, other calcium-rich foods or supplemental calcium are needed to meet your daily calcium requirement. In Chapter 9 we will discuss calcium in greater detail.

Table 5.4 Calcium content of protein-rich foods

Calcium rich protein food	Serving size	mg calcium/g protein
Milk	1 cup	300/8
Soy milk	1 cup	10/7
Soy milk (fortified)	1 cup	250/7
Tofu	4 oz	125/12
Tofu (fortified)	4 oz	250/12
Soy nuts	½ cup	225/20
Yogurt (plain)	1 cup	300/12
Swiss cheese	1 oz	250/8
Salmon (canned/bone)	4 oz	200/20
Sardines (whole)	4 oz	300/19
Whey protein	1 oz	30/20
Whey protein (fortified)	1 oz	250/20

Summary

Endurance athletes should consider the following key points regarding dietary protein intake:

- Research shows that for optimal performance and bone health your protein intake should be significantly higher than what is typically recommended.
- Endurance athletes should aim for 0.9–1.2 g of protein per pound of body weight per day. This level may need to be adjusted in response to training status, body composition, age, and overall diet quality.
- Certain whole-food protein sources may contain unique nutritional elements that are particularly helpful for endurance athletes. Examples are dairy products that have high calcium-to-protein ratios; whole soy foods that contain isoflavones; and cold-water fish that contain significant calcium (bone) as well as omega-3 fatty acids.
- Protein sources that are rich in the branched chain amino acids (isoleucine, leucine, valine) may be particularly important for endurance athletes as they appear to be important in maintaining the immune system and minimizing muscle damage.

■ Calcium excretion that is associated with protein intake may be offset by consuming a diet rich in alkalizing plant-based foods and ensuring adequate calcium intake.

REFERENCES

Amman P, Bourrin S, Bonjour J, Meyer J, Rizzoli R (2000) Protein under nutrition-induced bone loss is associated with decreased IGF-1 levels and estrogen deficiency. *Journal of Bone and Mineral Research* 15:683–690.

Bawa S (2010) The significance of soy protein and soy bioactive compounds in the prophylaxis and treatment of osteoporosis. *Journal of Osteoporosis* 2010 (8 pp.) (doi:10.4061/2010/891058).

Bigard A, Satabin P, Lavier P, Cannon F, Taillandier D, Guezennec C (1993) Effects of protein supplementation during prolonged exercise at moderate altitude on performance and plasma amino acid pattern. *European Journal of Physiology and Occupational Physiology* 66(1):5–10.

Bolster D, Pikosky M, Gaine P, Martin W, Wolfe R, Tipton K, Maclean D, Maresh C, Rodriquez N (2005) Dietary protein intake impacts human muscle protein fractional synthetic rates after endurance exercise. *American Journal of Physiology — Endocrinology and Metabolism* 289(4):E678–683.

Born S (2008) *The Endurance Athlete's Guide to Success, 8th Edition.* Whitefish, MT: Endurance, www.hammernutrition.com.

Breslau N, Brinkely L, Hill K (1988) Relationship of animal protein-rich diet to kidney stone formation and calcium metabolism. *Journal of Clinical Endocrinology and Metabolism* 66:140–146.

Coombes J, McNaughton L (2000) Effects of branched-chain amino acid supplementation of serum creatine kinase and lactate dehydrogenase after prolonged exercise. *Journal of Sports Medicine and Physical Fitness* 40:240–246.

Fenton T, Lyon A, Eliasziw M, Tough S, Hanley D (2009) Phosphate decreases urine calcium and increases calcium balance: a meta-analysis of the osteoporosis acid-ash diet hypothesis. *Nutrition Journal* 8:41 (doi:10.1186/1475-2891-8-41).

Fern E, Bielinski R, Schutz Y (1991) Effects of exaggerated amino acid and protein supply in man. *Experientia* 47:168–172.

Fielding R, Parkington J (2002) What are the dietary protein requirements of physically active individuals? New evidence on the effects of exercise on protein utilization during post exercise recovery. *Nutrition and Clinical Care* 5:191–196.

Forslund A, El-khoury EA, Olsson RM, Sjödin AM, Leif Hambraeus L, Young VRH (1999) Effect of protein intake and physical activity on 24-hour pattern and rate of macronutrient utilization. *American Journal of Physiology* 276:E964–E976.

Heaney R (2002) Protein and calcium: antagonists or synergists? *American Journal of Clinical Nutrition* 75:609–610.

Jamison N (2003) *Running Through The Wall.* Halcottsville, NY: Breakaway Books.

Kerstetter J, Svastisalee C, Caseria D, Mitnick M, Insogna K (2000) A threshold for low-protein-diet-induced elevations in parathyroid hormone. *American Journal of Clinical Nutrition* 72:168–173.

Koopman R, Pannemans D, Jeukendrup A, Gijsen A, Senden J, Halliday D, Saris W, van Loon L, Wagenmakers A (2004) Combined ingestion of protein and carbohydrate improves protein balance during ultra-endurance exercise. *American Journal of Physiology — Endocrinology and Metabolism* 287:E712–E720.

Lemon P, Dolny D, Yarasheski K (1997) Moderate physical activity can increase dietary protein needs. *Canadian Journal of Physiology* 22:494–503.

Massey L (2008) Does excess dietary protein adversely affect bone? Symposium overview. *The Journal of Nutrition* 128(6):1048–1050.

Messina M (2010) Soybean isoflavone exposure does not have feminizing effects on men: a critical examination of the clinical evidence. *Fertility and Sterility* 93(7):2095–2104.

Middleton N, Jelen P, Bell G (2004) Whole blood and mononuclear cell glutathione response to dietary whey protein supplementation in sedentary and trained male human subjects. *International Journal of Food and Science Nutrition* 55(2):131–141.

Negro M, Giardina S, Marzani B, Marzatico F (2008) Branched-chain amino acid supplementation does not enhance athletic performance but affects muscle recovery and the immune system. *Journal of Sports Medicine and Physical Fitness* 48(3):347–351.

Onywera V, Kiplamai F, Boit M, Pitsiladis Y (2005) Food and macronutrient intake of elite Kenyan distance runners. *International Journal of Sports Nutrition and Exercise Metabolism* 14(6):709–719.

Peters E (2003) Nutritional aspects in ultra-endurance exercise. *Current Opinion in Clinical Nutrition and Metabolic Care* 6(4):427–434.

Pikosky M, Smith T, Grediagin A, Castaneda-Sceppa C, Byerley L, Glickman E, Young A (2008) Increased protein maintains nitrogen balance during exercise induced energy deficit. *Medicine and Science in Sports and Exercise* 40(3):505–512.

Roughhead Z (2003) Is the interaction between dietary protein and calcium destructive or constructive for bone? Summary. *Journal of Nutrition* 133:866S–869S.

Tarnopolsky M, MacDougall J, Atkinson S (1998) Influence of protein intake and training status on nitrogen balance and lean body mass. *Journal of Applied Physiology* 64:187–193.

CHAPTER SIX

Dietary Fat

Dietary fat is a key energy source for endurance athletes because it provides nine calories per gram—more than twice as much as the four calories per gram provided by carbohydrates and proteins. Additionally, dietary fat plays a vital role in a multitude of body processes, including the absorption of certain nutrients (such as vitamin D) and the regulation of hormone levels and the immune system. As we have noted, diets containing moderate amounts of fat may have specific advantages for general health and thus reduce the likelihood of injury and improve endurance performance.

Dietary fats are classified as either *saturated* or *unsaturated*. Unsaturated fats can be further divided into *monounsaturated* or *poly-unsaturated* categories. The degree of saturation refers to the nature and structure of the chemical bonding that takes place between carbon and hydrogen atoms. In an unsaturated fat, each carbon atom is connected to the adjacent carbon atom with two chemical bonds, while in a saturated fat carbon atoms are connected to each other by single bonds, with the extra bonds used to link with extra hydrogen atoms. Therefore the term *hydrogenation* describes the process of chemically converting an unsaturated fat to one that is saturated by the addition of hydrogen atoms.

Historically, saturated fat has been linked with cardiovascular and many other degenerative diseases. More recently, researchers have determined that high levels of saturated fat also may compromise bone strength and lead to osteoporosis. For example, in 2006 Dr. Rebecca Corwin and her colleagues at The Pennsylvania State University reported that bone mineral density is inversely correlated with saturated fat intake. Males under 50 years old showed the greatest effects; the hip appeared to be the site that was most significantly influenced. Such studies are vitally important for endurance athletes who are considering experimenting with a higher fat diet. For the sake of your general health as well as performance, intake of saturated fat should continue to be limited. Foods that are high in saturated fat include prime-grade meats and whole-milk dairy products as well as lard, coconut, palm, and palm kernel oils.

Monounsaturated fats are considered "healthy fats" because they have been known to reduce total cholesterol levels and increase levels of HDL (good cholesterol). Monounsaturated fats recently have been found to improve bone quality and reduce fracture risk. Similarly, Martinez-Ramirez and colleagues (2007) discovered that study participants in the upper quartiles of polyunsaturated fatty acid (PUFA) intake showed an increased risk of sustaining an osteoporotic (low-energy) fracture while a protective effect was found in those individuals whose diets contained a higher ratio of monounsaturated fat (MUFA) to PUFA. Lastly, the overall intake of omega-6 fatty acids (common in some seeds, nuts, and their oils) was associated with an elevated risk of fracture.

Good sources of monounsaturated fats include avocados, olive oil, and some nuts. Nuts that contain the greatest percentage of monounsaturated fat include walnuts, macadamia nuts, pecans, pistachios, almonds, peanuts, and cashews.

Polyunsaturated fats have been shown to improve certain cardiovascular risk factors; for example, they do reduce total cholesterol. However, not all polyunsaturated fats are created equal. There are two major types of polyunsaturated fat that have received significant attention in both the scientific and popular press; omega-6 and omega-3. These two types of fats are considered essential because they cannot be synthesized by the body and therefore must be consumed in the diet. Omega-6 type fats are found in high concentrations in corn and safflower oils as well as processed foods made with vegetable oils. Excessive omega-6 intake has been associated with heart disease, cancer, and inflammation. Conversely, omega-3 fats have been demonstrated to promote good health in a multitude of ways, including reducing cardiovascular disease, total cholesterol, triglycerides, neuropsychiatric disorders (depression), and many inflammatory diseases (such as arthritis).

For endurance athletes interested in both performance and bone health, the news regarding omega-3 continues to get even better. For this information we thank Dr. Tim D. Mickleborough of Indiana University, whose original research underscores the connection between inflammation, performance, and health. His research group has demonstrated that a low-sodium diet (2005) reduces post-exercise-induced airway narrowing and moderates airway inflammation in asthmatic subjects. They also have demonstrated that a three-week fish oil diet, rich in omega-3 polyunsaturated fatty acids, has the protective effect of suppressing exercise-induced bronchoconstriction in both asthmatics (2006) and elite athletes (2003).

Omega-6 fatty acids precipitate inflammation and certain disease states whereas omega-3 fatty acids operate as anti-inflammatory agents. Dr. Mickleborough's respiratory research shows that high sodium intakes are also pro-inflammatory, so reducing salt intake improves endurance performance. Furthermore, by following a diet that is rich in anti-inflammatory omega-3 fatty acids, exercise capacity can be further enhanced.

You may wonder how these findings are related to skeletal health. Population studies establish that sodium intake in fact is correlated positively with inflammation (Fogarty, et al., 2009) and, in addition to compromising the respiratory system, high sodium intake appears to induce osteoporosis (Heaney, 2006). Sodium intake also correlates positively with calcium excretion and increases systemic inflammation to a degree that measurably reduces bone mass. In Chapter 7 we will further detail the specific pathways by which inflammation influences bone. At this stage it shouldn't surprise you to know that omega-3 fatty acid consumption leads to better bone quality (Lau, et al., 2009).

The main dietary sources of omega-3 fatty acids are cold water fatty fish (black cod, bluefish, herring, mackerel, salmon, and sardines), wild game, and supplemented eggs. Additional sources of omega-3 fatty acids include walnuts, flax seeds, and canola oil. Animal forms of omega-3 are considered superior to their plant-based counterparts.

The type of omega-3 most plentiful in plant form is known as *alpha-linolenic acid*, abbreviated ALA. In the body, ALA can be converted into longer chain forms including *docosahexaenoic acid* (DHA) and *eicosapentaenoic acid* (EPA). Unfortunately, during this conversion process less than 5% of ALA is turned into DHA. Consequently, most of the favorable biological effects on the body result from these longer forms that occur naturally in seafood and grass-fed animals. Intriguingly, one of the staples of the Mexican Tarahumara Indians, who are famous ultrarunners, is the chia seed (*Salvia hispanica*). The chia seed is an extremely rich source of plant type omega-3 fatty acids: a single ounce of seeds contains 4,915 mg (http://www.nutritionaldata.com/). The seed contains protein and fiber as well as many endurance-enhancing and bone-friendly minerals such as calcium and magnesium. Although we don't know if eating the chia seeds will give you the legendary endurance of the Tarahumara, based on the nutritional profile of these seeds they certainly appear to benefit both your general and your skeletal health!

For athletes to reap the many benefits of omega-3 fatty acids, leading authorities recommend consuming approximately 2 g per day. Additionally, a healthy ratio of omega-3 to omega-6 is considered necessary to maximize the health-enhancing benefits of these poly-unsaturated fats. A good ratio to strive for is a 1:2 or 1:3. This ratio means that for every gram of omega-3 that you consume, you should eat no more than 2–3 g of omega-6 (see Table 6.1).

It is very easy to damage polyunsaturated fats since their chem-ical composition renders them susceptible to molecular change when exposed to very high temperatures. Therefore, these fats should not be used for cooking, especially at high temperatures. For cooking purposes monounsaturated fats at low to medium temperatures are

Table 6.1 Common dietary sources of fatty acids

Sources of omega-3 fatty acids		
Food	Serving size	Omega-3 (g)
Wild salmon	3.5 oz	1–2
Sardines	3.5 oz	1–2
Mackerel	3.5 oz	1–2
Albacore Tuna	3.5 oz	1–2
Flax oil	1 tbsp	6.6
Flax seeds (ground)	1 tbsp	1.6
Soybeans	1 c	1.1
Walnuts	2 tbsp	1.0
Tofu	½ c	0.7
Leafy green vegetables	½ c	0.1

Sources of omega-6 fatty acids		
Food	Serving size	Omega-6 (g)
Safflower oil	1 tbsp	10.0
Sunflower oil	1 tbsp	9.0
Corn oil	1 tbsp	8.0
Soybean oil	1 tbsp	7.0

your best option. Extra-virgin olive oil is generally considered the gold standard cooking oil for its flavor, health benefits, and resistance to chemical alteration at low cooking temperatures.

Fat that has been chemically altered by processing is known as *trans-fat*. Trans-fatty acids are formed most frequently when liquid vegetable oils are converted into margarines or shortening by hydrogenation process. Consequently, a fatty acid described as being hydrogenated or partially hydrogenated contains trans-fat. These fats have been demonstrated to affect health negatively by altering blood lipid profiles and increasing inflammation.

The historical nutritional dogma has been that endurance athletes need to consume an abundant supply of carbohydrates and refrain from dietary fat. Unfortunately, this recommendation inadvertently may have undermined both skeletal and general health as well as limited the development of long-term endurance capacity. Stu Mittleman, an American record-holding and world-class ultrarunner, coach, and author, has shared his perspective on how his views of nutrition have changed over the course of his running career in his book *Slow Burn*. He writes,

> When I hear someone say that a food has fat in it, it means something totally different to me than it did fifteen years ago. Whereas once it meant that a particular food should be avoided, now I view fat as something that is indispensable to my diet. The main questions I want to answer are what type of fat is it and how much of it do I want. (pp. 232–233)

Summary

- In addition to their role as a fuel source, dietary fats help endurance athletes eliminate energy deficit, reduce injury risk, participate in the absorption of vitamin D, regulate hormone levels, and maintain their immune systems.

- Fats are broadly classified as being either saturated or unsaturated based on their chemical bonding characteristics. Saturated fats have been correlated with a number of degenerative conditions including cardiovascular disease and osteoporosis. Unsaturated fats are further classified as either monounsaturated or polyunsaturated. Monounsaturated fats, including olive oil and certain nuts, appear to support both general and bone health. The role of polyunsaturated fat intake is somewhat more complex.

- High-level intakes of the omega-6 variety of polyunsaturated fat appear to increase levels of systemic inflammation and a host of degenerative disorders including osteoporosis. By contrast, the omega-3 polyunsaturated fat reduces inflammation and enhances endurance performance.

- The recommendation for omega-3 intake per day is approximately 2 g.

- A 1:2 ratio of omega-3 to omega-6 is considered a good dietary standard for health and performance.

REFERENCES

Connor W, Cerqueira M, Connor R, Wallace R, Malinow M, Casdorph H (1978) The plasma lipids, lipoproteins, and diet of the Tarahumara Indians of Mexico. *The American Journal of Clinical Nutrition* 31:1131–1142.

Corwin R, Hartman T, Maczuga S, Graubard B (2006) Dietary saturated fat intake is inversely associated with bone density in humans: analysis of NHANES III. *Journal of Nutrition* 136(1):159–165.

Fogarty A, Lewis S, McKeever T, Britton J (2009) Is higher sodium intake associated with elevated systemic inflammation? A population-based study. *American Journal of Clinical Nutrition* 89(6):1901–1904.

Heaney R (2006) Role of dietary sodium in osteoporosis. *Journal of the American College of Nutrition.* 25(No. 90003):271S–276S.

Lau B, Ward W, Kang J, Ma D (2009) Vertebrae of developing fat-1 mice have greater strength and lower n-6/n-3 fatty acid ratio. *Experimental Biological Medicine (Maywood)* 234(6):632–638.

Martinez-Ramirez MJ, Palma S, Martinez-Gonzalez MA, Delgado-Martinez AD, de la Fuente C, Delgado-Rodriguez M (2007) Dietary fat intake and the risk of osteoporotic fractures in the elderly. *European Journal of Clinical Nutrition* 61(9):1114–1120.

Mickleborough T, Ionescu A, Lindley M, Fly A (2006) Protective effect of fish oil supplementation on exercise-induced bronchoconstriction in asthma. *Chest* 29(1):39–49.

Mickleborough T, Lindley M, Ray S (2005) Dietary salt, airway inflammation and diffusion capacity in exercise-induced asthma. *Medicine & Science in Sports & Exercise* 37(6):904–914.

Mickleborough T, Murray R, Ionescu A, Lindley M (2003) Fish oil supplementation reduces severity of exercise-induced bronchoconstriction in elite athletes. *American Journal of Respiratory Critical Care Medicine* 168(10):1181–1189.

Mittleman S, Callan K (2000) *Slow Burn*. New York: HarperCollins Publishers, Inc.

CHAPTER SEVEN

Inflammation

Inflammation is the immune system's mechanism of defense in response to injury, illness, or stress. The complex series of vascular and biochemical events, known collectively as the inflammatory response, is elicited when our physical or emotional health is threatened. A well-functioning immune system is necessary for survival and optimal health so that injuries can heal and invading organisms, such as viruses and bacteria, can be neutralized. Unfortunately, in certain situations, inflammation can become excessive and spread to involve all of the body's tissues, including bone. In addition to osteoporosis, we now know that other conditions are related to excessive inflammation, including insulin resistance, diabetes, irritable bowel syndrome, cardiovascular disease, food allergies, arthritis, some cancers, and nervous system disorders such as Alzheimer's disease.

Historically it has been recognized that moderate physical activity reduces illness rates relative to a sedentary lifestyle, but that prolonged or high-intensity exercise leads to increased risk of infection. This phenomenon is often described as being a "J-shaped model." Alternatively stated, a little exercise is good, and slightly more may be better, but beyond a certain degree, immunity is decreased, making athletes more susceptible to opportunistic diseases. For example, Nieman and colleagues examined 45 ultra distance runners competing in the Western States Endurance Run. They reported that of the 31 athletes who completed the 160-km race, 26% developed an upper respiratory tract infection within two weeks of completing the race.

William James wrote, "Beyond the very extreme of fatigue and distress, we may find amounts of ease and power we never dreamed ourselves to own; sources of strength never taxed at all because we never push through the obstruction." With this mantra as a guide, many athletes continue to push their physical and emotional boundaries in hopes of realizing their full potential. Unfortunately, many endurance athletes train and compete in a manner that supersedes their current level of preparedness. The results all too often are acute forms of injury or illness, as well as a chronically accelerated rate of degeneration. Additionally, many athletes are not aware of the interaction between the body's immune system and their nutritional practices; when the latter are poor, they ultimately may undermine not only their current performance level but also their long term health.

Physical Therapist and world class ultrarunner Scott Jurek was asked by interviewer George Beinhorn in *Trail Runner Magazine* (March 2007, trailrunnermagazine.com) about his vegan diet. The interviewer wanted to know: Can people become better trail runners by changing the way they eat? Scott Replied,

> You'll find people who have great diets and run pretty decently, and people who have very poor diets and run very fast. In terms of performance, diet may not help you on race day, but a healthy diet improves the body's ability to recover and repair. When you're young, you can bounce back quickly, but individuals who've paid attention to their diet for many years usually run and recover better later in life.

Following a strenuous training session or competition, several components of the immune system exhibit suppressed function. Respiratory tract infections or other similar conditions should not be ignored, as they often correlate with elevations of inflammatory markers. Altered states in the immune and inflammatory systems pose a challenge to health in general and bone health in particular.

It is quite possible that such overt signs of immune system compromise may be signaling enhanced bone turnover at a deeper level. Coaches, trainers, and athletes themselves should realize that prolonged training cycles, breakthrough training sessions, or an "A priority competition" need to be followed by a period of adequate rest and recovery. What is an appropriate "window" to allow for recovery and rebuilding of bone metabolism? There is no single formula here; rather, self-awareness and consultation with peers, a coach, or medical team is essential. An "easy" training day for an elite endurance athlete could produce a deep deficit for a recreational age grouper. To discover your own optimum performance criteria, maintaining a training log that includes information such as body weight, motivation, sleep quality, emotional state, resting heart rate, and results of finger tapping tests may be helpful in identifying deviations from the norm.

Elite endurance athletes either have worked hard to develop or innately possess the ability to recover quickly from hard efforts. This is one of the reasons they can accumulate training volumes and exercise intensities that propel them to the highest levels of human performance. However, as we will see, control of excessive inflammatory states and absorbing the benefits from training and competition may be as contingent upon lifestyle and training factors as genetics.

There simply is no single recovery formula that is best for all endurance athletes, so we recommend that you take the time to understand how your training, racing, and recovery may be related to the immune system. Although most of us are conditioned to believe that a "stronger" immune system is optimal the complex series of reactions that occurs in the body need to be well balanced in order to achieve both short and long term health. Age, experience, emotional state, and environmental considerations operate synergistically to influence immunity and therefore dictate an athlete's potential for exercise and recovery. The time for recovery and thus adaptation for any particular athlete is unique. This physiological diversity is especially important for teams to consider as often workouts are not individualized. Recovery is contingent upon the influence that the immune system has over the multitude of an athlete's systems (nervous, articular, psychological, cardiovascular, endocrine, metabolic, musculoskeletal); any of these may be a rate limiting factor for a given athlete.

To understand why recovery following the same ultramarathon may be so variable, consider the training and level of preparedness between two former patients. The first athlete averaged 60–75 running miles per week for the last three years, and was a former track and collegiate crosscountry athlete. He included specific hill workouts twice per week for the preceding three months. In addition, he included three training sessions in which he ran parts of the actual race course in order to familiarize himself with the technical demands and footing. He has experimented and developed a successful strategy for carbohydrate, fluid, and electrolyte replacement under different environmental conditions. Additionally, he has spent extensive time cultivating his running technique, muscle, and connective tissue elasticity, as well as emotional balance through thoughtful physical training methods and meditation.

In contrast, the second competitor had run intermittently in the past, but never competitively, and for the nine months before the race averaged 25–30 miles per week. He had never completed a single run that exceeded 18 miles within the past three months. Moreover, he relied on the aid stations at the race to supply his fuel and had never experimented with the particular sports drink that was to be supplied.

Following the ultramarathon, the first runner observed a slight increase in resting heart rate as well as a reduced number of finger taps per minute, indicating a generalized stress reaction and central nervous system inhibition. Additionally, a mild general stiffness affected his lower extremity muscles and reduced the muscles' ability to generate force and/or efficiently relax. His physical symptoms had returned to baseline within five days and he developed no infections. His emotional state was slightly depressed for the 48 hours immediately following the race as he felt somewhat "depleted." As these feelings resolved, he felt a sense of accomplishment as he became more aware that his potential was realized to its highest level to date and that his preparation was consistent with the demands of the race.

The second competitor reported extensive muscle and connective tissue soreness, knee swelling, and sharp localized pain in the heels. He was physically exhausted but felt emotionally anxious and was unable to sleep well. Carbohydrate cravings, dry mouth, and diarrhea persisted for several days. Upper respiratory track infection developed within two days following the race and persisted for nearly two weeks. He felt as though he never wanted to return to running again.

The point of drawing this contrast is not to encourage all runners to average 75 miles per week over hard courses to be ready for the "big race" whenever it comes. Rather, we stress here the critical importance of knowing realistically one's individual level of conditioned ability. A fair recommendation for training is to consider workouts that you cannot recover from within 24 hours as being excessive for your particular level of ability. Making a habit of engaging in training or racing that frequently crosses this threshold is a recipe for the development of perturbations in the multiple systems that are necessary for overall and bone health.

We often are able to discuss with injured athletes, particularly adult recreational marathon runners, the events that led to their stress fractures. Many of these individuals are relatively new to running and had been running for less than a year when they decided to train for their first marathon. Rarely were they running more than three times per week for more than 30–45 minutes in each session prior to embarking on a marathon training program printed in a popular running magazine. Their 12-week generic training regimen consisted of running two or three "short" runs during the week, with a progressively longer run on the weekend. The longer run often was more than 50–60% of their total weekly running mileage. Many reported that they noticed mild pain in the exact location of what eventually would be diagnosed as a stress fracture at the end of their longest training run. Because they tapered off training for the next several weeks following their single "long" training run, the pain disappeared and was undetectable by the start of the marathon. Unfortunately, around the half-marathon distance, the former pain reappeared. By mile 20, severe pain prevented further running, and they were forced to walk. Following the race, at the medical tent, they were diagnosed with "shin splints" or a probable stress fracture.

Independently, many relatively high volume runners who have had stable running backgrounds develop a stress fracture later in life for "no apparent reason." After diagnosis, they learn that their bone mass is well below age expected norms for their ages, and they wonder how this has occurred. Because of the absence of symptoms associated with osteoporosis, these individuals were unaware that their skeletons were losing bone. In the next section we will detail some of the inflammatory pathways that directly influence bone, and then suggest some nutritional countermeasures.

Inflammation and Bone

Athletes often are surprised to learn that the immune system modulates skeletal health. Bone remodeling occurs through the actions of protein or hormonal messengers known as *cytokines*. Collectively cytokines balance bone remodeling by exerting either pro- or anti-inflammatory actions that directly influence osteoclasts and osteoblasts. The principal messengers involved in the inflammatory-bone interactions are known as RANK, RANKL, and OPG. Expanding these acronyms, respectively, we have RANK (receptor activator of nuclear factor KB), RANKL (a *ligand* of RANK, a ligand being a substance that binds to another molecule and serves as a trigger signaling mechanism), and OPG (osteoprotegrin, which inhibits the production of osteoclasts). Briefly, then, RANK and RANK-L are osteoclast activators and OPG (osteoprotegerin) is an inhibitor. When inflammatory reactions are elevated, RANKL predominates over OPG, and bone loss ensues.

In addition to these inflammatory pathways, the body's immune response also includes numerous other cytokines that exert direct and indirect influences over bone. Interleukin-6 (IL-6) is one such additional chemical messenger that modifies osteoclast maturation; IL-6 is of special interest for athletes because recent research indicates that it is released by skeletal muscle contractions during exercise (Pederson, 2009). In response to decreased estrogen levels or calcium availability, Interleukin-1 and Interleukin-8 (IL-1, IL-8) are known to activate osteoclasts, resulting in enhanced bone loss. Other cytokines also are known to regulate bone cell activity; according to Ding, et al. (2008) and Mcean (2009), these include nitric oxide (NO) and tumor necrosis factor alpha (TNF-α).

Overtraining and Inflammation

Overtraining is associated with a variety of signs and symptoms that may be hard to define objectively. However, when an athlete is training or competing in a manner that exceeds his or her capacity for emotional or physical recovery, a state of overreaching or overtraining is said to exist. One way in which exercise scientists attempt to objectively determine an athlete's physiologic state is by evaluating the ratio of reproductive (estrogen) or anabolic (testosterone) to catabolic (cortisol) hormone levels, as well as measuring markers of muscle damage or inflammation.

In 2008 Neubauer and colleagues studied the blood chemistry of 42 male triathletes two days before, immediately after, then one, five, and 19 days following an Ironman distance triathlon. Blood samples were analyzed for a variety of inflammatory markers, hormones, and muscle damage. Results demonstrated that immediately following the race there were increases in total leukocyte counts, MPO (myeloperoxidase, whose breakdown products kill bacteria), PMN elastase (a proteolytic enzyme that is raised in response to inflammation and sepsis), cortisol, CK (creatine kinase) activity, myoglobin, IL-6, IL-10 (cytokines that act as mediators among leucocytes and are important in the immune response), and hs-CRP (high sensitivity C-reactive protein). At the same time, testosterone levels measurably decreased. Most of these disturbances returned to baseline within one day following the race, but a low-grade systemic inflammation persisted for over five days. While it will come as no surprise that endurance events can be stressful, many athletes do not realize that the negative effects, and thus recovery needs, can last for weeks or even months.

In addition to self-monitoring and maintaining a training log, we also suggest that athletes consider having an annual consultation with a primary care or sports medicine physician. The examination might well include blood tests for both anabolic and catabolic hormones as well as tests for systemic inflammation. The most common means for determining systemic inflammation levels is a C reactive protein (hs-CRP) test.

CRP is a blood protein that is formed in the liver and released in response to inflammation-inducing events; it also is thought to play a role in innate immunity. Normal concentrations in healthy adults are less than 10 mg/L. Slightly elevated levels also commonly arise during pregnancy and minor viral infections (10–40 mg/L). CRP levels may be increased by 50,000 fold during the time of an active or severe infection. Although CRP is a non-specific marker of inflammation, it commonly is used for medical screening purposes as its elevated levels have been linked to pain, arthritis, diabetes, hypertension, cardiovascular disease, and cancer (Haheim, et al., 2009).

Free Radicals and Inflammation

Free radical mechanisms have been implicated in many of the same degenerative conditions that are known to accompany excessive inflammation, including osteoporosis. Free radicals are unstable molecules that interact with various body tissues in an attempt to improve electrical stability by "borrowing" available electrons. Affected body tissues include cell membranes, proteins, lipids, and DNA. The cellular damage that results from this electron exchange induces the release of pro-inflammatory cytokines, leading to bone loss. The free radical theory has a broad scope beyond bone biology alone, proposing that lifespan is inversely related to metabolic rate and thus oxygen consumption.

The human body possesses antioxidation mechanisms that prevent or reduce free radical damage. These metabolic activities are dependent upon the presence of certain nutritional factors. Substances commonly considered to be antioxidants include vitamins C and E, as well as beta-carotene (a precursor of Vitamin A). Many other nutritional factors, including coenzyme Q10 (a helper molecule that is part of the electron transport chain that functions in aerobic metabolism), are known to provide background support as well as being involved in the recycling of antioxidants.

In 2006 Dr. W.L. Knez and colleagues from the University of Queensland published a paper in the *Sports Medicine Journal*, including the finding that at least 30 minutes of moderate-intensity physical activity (accumulated most, and preferably all) days should be considered the minimum level necessary to reduce the risk of developing cardiovascular disease.

Despite an unknown underlying mechanism, some epidemiological data paradoxically suggest that a very high volume of exercise is associated with a *decrease* in cardiovascular health. Although, as we have noted earlier, moderate endurance exercise training has been shown to decrease inflammation and increase antioxidant defenses (and therefore confer a protective effect against oxidative stress), excessive oxidative stress may contribute to the development of atherosclerosis via oxidative modification of low-density lipoprotein (LDL).

Research also has shown that endurance exercise can be associated with acute cardiac dysfunction and injury, possibly due to an increase in free radical production. Longitudinal studies are needed to assess whether antioxidant defenses are adequate to prevent LDL oxidation that may occur as a result of increased free radical production during very high volumes or intensities of exercise.

It is highly likely that some of the negative effects of oxidative stress can be offset by dietary antioxidants. The USDA Food and Nutrition Center (FNIC) of the National Agricultural Library (NAL) have provided a list of foods that are among the best sources of dietary antioxidants:

Artichoke

Apples (gala, granny smith, red delicious)

Beans (black, kidney, pinto, small red)

Blackberry

Blueberries (wild and cultivated)

Cranberry

Pecan

Plums (black and other varieties)

Prune

Raspberry

Russet Potato

Strawberry

Sweet Cherry

Nutrition and Inflammation

Historically sports nutrition experts have emphasized the value of adequate caloric intake and carbohydrate availability to maximize performance. Recent nutritional research indicates that food selection may play an important role in modulation of systemic inflammation and thus health and performance. Some foods are considered pro-inflammatory. These include refined grains, some processed and packaged foods, high glycemic foods, trans-fats, and grain-fed meats. In contrast, we just have seen that some foods that are high in natural antioxidants that are likely to help in reducing inflammation. Foods considered anti-inflammatory include fruits, vegetables, fish, legumes, tea, and grass- or pasture-fed meat. Additionally, certain spices including turmeric and ginger have been demonstrated to have anti-inflammatory properties.

Recent research tested the effects of ginger on exercise induced muscle pain and soreness. In one study, subjects consumed 2 g (roughly one teaspoon) of either raw or heat treated ginger seven days prior and three days following a session of eccentric weight lifting (three sets of six repetitions with a weight equal to 120% of the concentric 1RM). Results were impressive, with the ginger trials resulted in 25% (raw) and 23% (heat treated) less muscle pain and soreness compared to the placebo (Black, et al., 2010).

In another study of 60 adults aged 18–50 years, those who drank 10.5 ounces of cherry juice twice a day for seven days prior to and on the day of a long distance running relay had significantly less pain following the race than those who drank another fruit juice beverage. On a scale from zero to 10, the runners who drank cherry juice as their "sports drink" had a two point lower self-reported pain level at the completion of the race, a clinically significant difference (Kuehl, et al., 2009).

Similarly, in the London Marathon Study on Tart Cherry Juice, conducted the same year, 20 subjects (13 men) were randomly assigned to take cherry juice or placebo. The drinks were given twice a day for five days prior to the marathon race, on the day of the race (one pre, one post) and for two days after the race. Blood samples were taken prior to supplementation, on the day prior to the race, immediately following the race, and one and two days post race. Samples were analyzed for total antioxidant capacity (TAC), markers of muscle damage (CK, LDH), inflammation (IL-6, CRP, uric acid), and oxidative stress. Additionally, isometric knee extension strength and muscle soreness were assessed on the evening prior to the race and one and two days post race. The results showed that total anti-oxidant capacity increased by 11% in the cherry juice group with no change being detected in the placebo group. In the cherry juice group, Il-6 elevation was 49% lower, and CRP elevation was 34% lower than placebo. Strength loss immediately after the race was similar between groups (cherry juice 76% of baseline, placebo 73% of baseline) but the cherry juice group showed a more rapid recovery of strength (90% on Day 1 and 101% on Day 2) compared with placebo (81% on Day 1 and 91% on Day 2). See McHugh and Howatson (2008). Beyond these featured studies, there also have been several broader investigations of nutrition-inflammation interactions (Calder, et al., 2009; Cavicchia, et al., 2009; Pan, et al., 2009).

Potassium and Magnesium

Nutrition-inflammation mechanisms are complex and so contingent upon a variety of factors that no single food or supplement provides immunity from inflammatory induced bone loss. However, potassium and magnesium are minerals that appear to be particularly important in the modulation of inflammation.

Many individuals have diets low in potassium, with population studies often revealing intakes in the 2,000–3,000 mg range, while the DRI (Daily Recommended Intake by the USDA) for potassium is currently set at 4,000 mg. For example, Zalcman and colleagues (2007) evaluated the nutritional intakes of ultra-endurance adventure racers and reported that "For most vitamins and minerals, athletes' intake was adequate, with the exception of magnesium, zinc, and potassium in men and vitamin E and calcium in women, which presented a high probability of being inadequate compared to reference values."

Low potassium diets also result in an inflammatory state as well as impairments of glucose utilization and glycogen storage. Endurance athlete also may appreciate knowing that low potassium levels have been associated with impaired blood flow during exercise (Young, et al., 1995).

In addition to the important role potassium plays in exercise metabolism, it also is a key element for the regulation of body pH (for more detail on this topic, see Acid/Base Regulation). Intense exercise leads to decreases in pH that require buffering from ingested food. Foods that contain potassium exert an alkalinizing effect by generating potassium bicarbonate. The following list of potassium levels in select foods is developed from the USDA National Nutrient Database and Hands (2000):

Fruits
Cantaloupe (1 c) 427 mg
Bananas (1) 422 mg
Pears (1) 333 mg
Mangoes (1) 323 mg
Apple (1) 150 mg
Orange (1) 150

Vegetables

Tomatoes (1 c) 528 mg

Broccoli (1 cup) 400 mg

Baby carrots (1) 24 mg

Dried fruit

Raisins (1/2 cup) 600 mg

Apricots (1/2 cup) 900 mg

Figs (1/2 cup) 700 mg

Meat and fish

Chicken breast (1) 500 mg

Cod fillet (1) 450 mg

Steak (3 oz) 300 mg

Dietary magnesium insufficiency may influence the body's inflammatory state via aerobic metabolic pathways. This mineral is involved in adenosine triphosphaste (ATP) production via fatty acid oxidation (aerobic metabolism). Consequently, magnesium deficiency may result in compromised mitochondrial function and increased free radical formation. In addition, magnesium deficiency appears to trigger a cascade of events that is initiated by the release of *Substance P,* a neurotransmitter associated with pain; the result is increased production of both immune cells and pro-inflammatory cytokines.

Low magnesium levels can cause acute symptoms of fatigue, nausea, and muscle cramps while chronic deficiency has been linked with anemia and osteoporosis. The current recommended levels of daily intake for magnesium are:

Adolescent females, 360 mg

Adolescent males, 410 mg

Adult females, 320 mg

Adult males, 420 mg

Population-based studies of athletes and non-athletes reveal that typical intakes of magnesium are either adequate or slightly insufficient. A 1999 report on the diets of female athletes engaged in a variety of sports (karate, handball, basketball, and running) revealed that no group of athletes reached the minimal daily intake for magnesium or zinc, although their values were superior to that of the control group (Nuviala, et al., 1999). For excellent reviews on the topic of magnesium in the context of exercise and immune function, see Konig, et al. (1998) as well as Shephard and Shek (1998). The following list of magnesium levels in select foods was drawn from the USDA Nutrient Database:

Fruit
Banana (1 medium) 101 mg
Dried Figs (4) 44 mg

Vegetables
Artichoke (1 c) 101 mg
Spinach, cooked (1 c) 157 mg
Broccoli, frozen (1 c) 37 mg
Beet greens (1 c) 98 mg
Summer squash (1 c) 43 mg

Beans, lentils
Black beans (1 c) 81 mg
Navy beans (1 c) 107 mg
Lentils (1 c) 71 mg
Chickpeas (1 c) 79 mg

Nuts, seeds
Almonds (2 oz) 156 mg
Brazil nuts (2 oz) 128 mg
Cashews (2 oz) 148 mg
Pumpkin seeds (1 oz) 151 mg

Grains
Brown rice (1 c) 84 mg
Whole wheat flour (1 c) 166 mg
Pearled barley, raw (1 c) 158 mg
Oat bran, raw (1 c) 221 mg

Blood Glucose Control

Traditionally, endurance athletes have been advised to eat a high carbohydrate diet (carbohydrates greater than 60% of calories) for both performance and health. This recommendation may need to be reconsidered. Because endurance trained individuals exhibit low levels of triglycerides, it has been assumed that this favorable state is a *chronic* adaptation to exercise participation. However, this state is rapidly reversed in the absence of training, so it is likely that the triglyceride lowering effects of exercise are mainly the result of *acute* metabolic responses to recent exercise rather than long-term training adaptations, per se.

In 2006 Kopp published the review paper "The atherogenic potential of dietary carbohydrate" in the *Preventive Medicine Journal*. The results of the review showed that high carbohydrate nutrition has the ability to induce vascular inflammation and plaque formation through an insulin-mediated activation of the renin-angiotensin system (RAS), growth factors, cytokines, the sympathetic nervous system, and C-reactive protein. The interaction causes an atherogenic lipid profile in normal humans. Epidemiologic investigations as well as studies in experimental animals corroborate an important role of dietary carbohydrates in atherogenesis. The strong implication of this study is that high carbohydrate diets, particularly in the form of high-glycemic index or manufactured carbohydrates, have the ability to directly induce atherosclerosis and the same inflammatory pathways known to adversely influence bone. It was suggested that the reason for these dietary-induced, insulin-mediated, atherogenic metabolic perturbations is an insufficient adaptation to starch and sugars during human evolution. Restriction of insulinogenic foods (starches and sugars) may help to prevent the development of atherosclerosis one of the most common and costliest human diseases. Kopp's suggestion is that it may be metabolically safe to consume a diet that is high in carbohydrate only while engaged in enough exercise to offset its detrimental effects on pro-inflammatory cytokines and triglyceride levels.

There now is sufficient evidence that diets more moderate in carbohydrate (40%) and higher in fat (30–40%) enable the endurance athlete to both perform well and reduce the likelihood of developing an inflammatory metabolic state. For additional reading on the topic of diet induced inflammation we recommend the following articles: Leddy, et al. (1997); Thompson, et al. (1984); Brown and Cox (1998); Hellerstein (2002); Gill and Hardman (2003); Geraldo and Alfenas (2008); Levitan, et al. (2008).

Athletes concerned about the likelihood of adverse events associated with straying away from the typically recommended high-carbohyrdrate low-fat training diet should read an article by Venkatraman and colleagues (1995). They recognized that athletes are competitive, train at very high levels with inadequate rest, consume too few calories, avoid fats, and may be at increased risk of infections. Since the immune system is sensitive to both fat intake and intense exercise, athletes may have suppressed immune function resulting from imbalances between diet and exercise. Many athletes consume about 25% fewer calories than estimated expenditure, leading to low intakes of some essential micronutrients and fats. While chronic participation in moderate exercise may help reduce systemic inflammation, prolonged or intense training and racing has been shown to increase inflammatory immune factors, decrease anti-inflammatory ones, and increase oxidant stress.

Because lipids are powerful mediators of the immune system, they may modulate the immunosuppressive effects of strenuous exercise. Studies have shown that a low-fat, high-carbohydrate diet (15% fat, 65% CHO, 20% protein of total calories) of the sort typically eaten by athletes can have negative effects. These outcomes include increases in inflammatory and decreases in anti-inflammatory immune factors, depression of anti-oxidants, and negative influences on blood lipoprotein ratios. Increasing caloric intake by 25% to match energy expenditure, and increasing dietary fat intake to 32%, appears to reverse the negative effects on immune function and lipoprotein levels reported for athletes on a low-fat diet. Increasing the dietary fat intake of athletes to 42%, while maintaining caloric intake equal to expenditure, does not negatively affect immune competency or blood lipoproteins. This higher energy, higher fat regimen has been shown to improve endurance exercise performance at 60–80% of VO2 max in cyclists, soldiers, and runners.

Although there may be times when an endurance athlete consumes a high carbohydrate meal, such as immediately following exhaustive exercise, a steady intake of highly refined carbohydrates, devoid of fruits and vegetables seems undesirable for general and skeletal health. In the various chapters we will provide suggestions on what to eat before, during, and after exercise as well as provide more detail on dietary carbohydrate, fat, and protein.

Summary

Endurance athletes who are interested in reducing inflammation and thus bone loss should consider the following recommendations:

- Maintain adequate energy balance.
- Consume abundant fruits and vegetables.

- Include teas and spices known to have potent anti-inflammatory effects.

- Consider foods rich in potassium and magnesium as being particularly important for endurance and bone health.

- Reduce or eliminate inflammation-producing foods including highly refined manufactured foods or those containing trans fats.

- Seek to maintain stable levels of blood glucose by balancing carbohydrate ingestion with adequate dietary protein and fat and/or eliminating the consumption of highly refined carbohydrate sources.

REFERENCES

Black C, Herring M, Hurley D, O'Connor P (2010, in press) Ginger (*Zingiber officinale*) reduces muscle pain caused by eccentric exercise. *The Journal of Pain* (doi: 10.1016/j.jpain.2009.12.013).

Brown R, Cox C (1998) Effects of high fat versus high carbohydrate diets on plasma lipids and lipoproteins in endurance athletes. *Medicine and Science in Sports and Exercise* 30(12):1677–1683.

Calder P, et al. [21 authors] (2009) Inflammatory disease processes and interactions with nutrition. *British Journal of Nutrition* May, 101 Suppl. 1:S1–45.

Cavicchia PP, Steck SE, Hurley TG, Hussey JR, Ma Y, Ochene IS, Hebert JR (2009) A new dietary inflammatory index predicts interval changes in serum high-sensitivity C-reactive protein. *Journal of Nutrition* 139(12):2365–2372.

Ding C, Parameswaran V, Udayan R, Burgess J, Jones G (2008) Circulating levels of inflammatory markers predict change in bone mineral density and resorption in older adults: a longitudinal study. *Journal of Clinical Endocrinology & Metabolism* 93(5):1952–1958.

Febbraio, MA (2007) Exercise and inflammation. *Journal of Applied Physiology* 103:376–377.

Geraldo J, Alfenas R (2008) Role of diet on chronic inflammation prevention and control-current evidences. *Arquivos Brasileiros Endocrinologia & Metabologia* 52(6):951–967.

Gill JMR, Hardman AE (2003) Exercise and postprandial lipid metabolism: an update on potential mechanisms and interactions with high carbohydrate diets (review). *The Journal of Nutritional Biochemistry* 14(3):122–132.

Haheim L, Nafstad P, Olsen I, Schwarze P, Ronningen K (2009) C-reactive protein variations for different chronic somatic disorders. *Scandinavian Journal of Public Health* 37(6):640–646.

Hands ES (2000) *Nutrients in Food*. Philadelphia: Lippincott Williams & Wilkins.

Hellerstein M (2002) Carbohydrate-induced hypertriglyceridemia: modifying factors and implications for cardiovascular risk. *Current Opinion in Lipidology* 13(1):33–40.

Knez W, Coombes J, Jenkins D (2006) Ultra-endurance exercise and oxidative damage: implications for cardiovascular health. *Sports Medicine* 36(5): 429–441.

Konig D, Weinstock C, Keul J, Northhoff H, Berg A (1998) Zinc, iron, and magnesium status in athletes-influences on the regulation of exercise-induced stress and immune function. *Exercise Immunology Review* 4:2–21.

Kopp W (2006) The atherogenic potential of dietary carbohydrate. *Prevenitve Medicine* 42(5):336–342.

Kuehl K, Chestnutt J, Elliot D (May, 2009) Efficacy of tart cherry juice in reducing muscle pain after strenuous exercise. *Journal of the International Society of Sports Nutrition* 7:17. Published online 2010 May 7. doi: 10.1186/1550-2783-7-17.

Leddy J, Horvath P, Rowland J, Pendergast D (1997) Effect of a high or low fat diet on cardiovascular risk factors in male and female runners. *Medicine and Science in Sports and Exercise* 29(1):17–25.

Levitan E, Cook N, Stampfer M, Ridker P, Rexrode K, Buring J, Manson J, Liu S (2008) Dietary glycemic index, dietary glycemic load, blood lipids, and C-reactive protein. *Metabolism* 57(3):437–443.

McHugh MP, Howatson G (2008) Summary Report on the Cherrypharm 2008 London Marathon Study. Report submitted to Cherrypharm on July 22, 2008 (see *New England Runner*, www.runtohomebse.org).

Mcean R (2009) Proinflammatory cytokines and osteoporosis. *Current Osteoporosis Reports* 74(4):134–139.

Neubauer O, Konig D, Wagner KH (2008) Recovery after an Ironman triathlon: sustained inflammatory responses and muscular stress. *European Journal of Applied Physiology* 104(3):417–426.

Nieman D, Dumke C, Henson D, McAnulty S, McAnulty L, Lind R, Morrow J (2003) Immune and oxidative changes during and following the Western States Endurance Run. *International Journal of Sports Medicine* 24(7): 541–547.

Nuviala R, Lapieza M, Bernal E (1999) Magnesium, zinc, and copper status in women involved in different sports. *International Journal of Sports Nutrition* 9(3):295–309.

Pan MH, Lai CS, Dushenkov S, Ho C (2009) Modulation of inflammatory genes by natural dietary bioactive compounds. *Journal of Agricultural and Food Chemistry* 57:4467–4447.

Pederson B (2009) Edward F. Adolph distinguished lecture: muscle as an endocrine organ: IL-6 and other myokines. *Journal of Applied Physiology* 107(4):1006–1014.

Shephard R, Shek P (1998) Immunological hazards from nutritional imbalances in athletes. *Exercise Immunology Review* 4:22–48.

Thompson P, Cullinane E, Eshleman R, Kantor M, Herbert P (1984) The effects of high-carbohydrate and high-fat diets on the serum lipid and lipo-protein concentrations of endurance athletes. *Metabolism* 33(11):1003–1010.

Venkatraman J, Leddy J, Pendergast D (1995) Dietary fats and immune status in athletes: clinical implications. *Medicine and Science in Sports and Exercise* 32(7):S389–S395.

Young D, Lin H, McCabe R (1995) Potassium's cardiovascular protective mechanism. *American Journal of Physiology* 268:R825–R837.

Zalcman I, Guarita H, Juzwiak C, Crispim C, Antunes H, Edwards B, Tufik S, De Mello M (2007) Nutritional status of adventure racers. *Nutrition* 23(5):404–411.

CHAPTER EIGHT

Acid-Base Regulation

Endurance exercise can present serious challenges to the maintenance of normal pH, and in turn abnormal pH levels can accelerate calcium loss and consequently damage bone health. In physiology, electrolytes that release hydrogen ions (H+) are considered acids and substances that readily combine with hydrogen ions are considered bases. The concentration of hydrogen ions in the body is expressed in pH units, which measure "potential of Hydrogen" on a scale of zero to 14. Normal arterial blood pH at rest is approximately 7.4 ± 0.02 and maintenance of this normal range is extremely important as deviations influence the rate at which many metabolic processes occur, including the rate at which the skeleton remodels.

Traditionally, it was assumed that the increase in hydrogen ion concentration was a cause of fatigue arising from increases in lactic acid. This classic explanation of fatigue has been in place for nearly 100 years, but significant evidence now refutes the model. Many studies demonstrate that although lactic acid is increased, this increase in itself does not limit exercise capacity; in fact, it actually may be necessary to sustain performance.

Metabolic *acidosis* during exercise is related to reactions other than lactate production. Every time ATP is degraded during exercise metabolism, a proton is released. When exercise is steady state and ATP demand can be matched via mitochondrial oxidative mechanisms (aerobic energy metabolism), there is no net accumulation of hydrogen ions. However, when exercise intensity is increased and ATP demand exceeds oxidative capacity, there is a net increase in hydrogen ion concentration and a corresponding reduction in pH. During intense exercise, pH levels are decreased to as low as 7.0.

pH Range of Arterial Blood
(Acidosis) 7.0 ← 7.4 → 7.8 (Alkalosis)

During high-intensity endurance exercise, muscle and blood pH decrease due to the rise in production of hydrogen ion via anaerobic energy systems of energy production. The intensity at which pH starts to decline is generally in the order of 50–60% VO2 max (the maximum volume of oxygen that can be utilized in one minute of intense exercise). Although the reduction in pH is known to be related to the net accumulation of hydrogen ion concentration (rather than to lactate specifically), lactate concentrations act as an excellent marker of pH alterations as changes in lactate parallel changes in body pH. Lactate levels in the resting state are measured on the order of 1 mMol/L and can increase as much as 20 fold during sustained high intensity exercise efforts.

During a graduated exercise test, acidity levels increase (as measured by declines in pH) commensurate with effort. Historically, there has been a reference point during a test that has been described as the "anaerobic or lactate threshold." This point has been considered the effort level at which exercise metabolism switches from primarily aerobic to anaerobic. Today, most exercise scientists agree that there is not a discrete intensity level at which this cross over from primarily aerobic to anaerobic metabolism occurs. However, it still is a useful concept to consider when discussing training or racing efforts. As a functional guide, this exercise intensity level is generally field tested as the maximal speed (or power) that can be maintained for a 12–24 minute time trial. Many runners use their fastest 5K distance and many rowers use a 20 minute time trial to determine this exercise intensity. With training, this speed or power is increased relative to an athlete's maximal aerobic capacity (VO2 max). For many athletes, this "lactate threshold intensity" corresponds to approximately 85% of their maximal aerobic capacity. However, as fitness improves, athletes can perform at a higher percentage of their maximal capacity (VO2 max). In other words, their anaerobic or lactate threshold increases relative to a stable VO2 max. Although maximal aerobic capacity is known to be favorably correlated with the likelihood of success in endurance activities, the percentage of this maximum that an athlete can sustain is a better predictor of actual performance. Elite athletes are capable of working at very high percentages of their maximal aerobic capacity for prolonged periods.

One of the earliest recorded field studies demonstrating this was performed by Dr. Joan Ullyot, MD (1978). In this observational analysis, Dr. Ullyot monitored 1968 Olympian marathoner Ron Daws' heart rate for the duration of a marathon in which he finished in 2:26:58. Ron's heart rate stayed between 177 and 180 beats per minute for the duration of the race. This level of heart rate corresponded to approximately 95% of his maximum heart rate of 187 beats per minute as determined by an exhaustive treadmill test.

We recommend that endurance athletes consider utilizing a standard time or distance trial (20 minute time trial, 5–6K distance trial) throughout the training year to assess changes in fitness. As fitness improves, speed (or power) is known to increase without increases in blood lactate or reductions in pH. Alternatively stated, you will be moving faster in a more efficient manner. For those coaches or athletes who monitor lactate levels, this is known as shifting the lactate curve to the right. Common exercise strategies to induce the rightward shift include "pushing" or "pulling" the lactate threshold. Pushing the curve refers to building up the exercise volume on the left side of the existing curve, while pulling involves the performance of higher intensity exercise efforts that exceed that of the existing curve.

When a state of relative acidosis exists in the body, there is an associated increase in urine calcium excretion that may lead to a net calcium loss. Because the skeleton is the body's primary calcium storage site, the source of the calcium excretion is considered to most likely be from bone. High intensity endurance exercise that creates a metabolic acidosis favors both increases in osteoclastic resorption as well as reductions in osteoblastic formation.

In 2002 Dressendorfer and colleagues studied the effects of a periodized program of intense endurance training on basal plasma and 24-hour urinary excretion of key minerals in competitive male cyclists (n = 9). The training consisted of a six-week volume phase in which average training intensity was 87% of maximal heart rate, an interval phase lasting 18 days during which training intensity was 100% of heart rate max, and a 10-day unloading taper. Compared to the baseline, performance improved significantly, while mineral metabolism was not significantly different after the volume phase. However, after the interval phase, renal calcium excretion was increased and plasma calcium fell slightly below the clinical norm. Other minerals including magnesium, iron, zinc, and copper metabolism remained unchanged throughout the study (Dressendorfer, et al., 2002).

The type of exercise stress that is known to result in the greatest degree of acidosis results from effort that is performed above the so-called lactate threshold point for greater than one to two minutes. The racing events that induce the greatest alteration in pH is rowing 2000 meters, running middle distances (800 meters, mile), or "breaking away" from the pack on the bike. These are situations that require near maximal efforts be maintained for extended periods of time.

Energy Systems

Perhaps no greater summary of exercise metabolism exists than the one provided by the late George Sheehan, MD, who wrote in his famous book *Running and Being,*

> The runner has three great challenges, and the greatest of these is the mile. The others are the dash and the marathon. Taken together, they comprise all of exercise physiology. They correspond to the three major sources of muscular energy, and they call on man in his various guises as body, mind, and spirit. The dash is raw speed powered by high-energy phosphates. The marathon is the unerring test of endurance and the use of oxygen. But the mile is all these, plus a third force, anaerobic metabolism, the use of sugar in the absence of oxygen, and the ability to clear the body of lactic acid.

Classic exercise physiology texts describe human energy production as stemming from three distinct pathways: *anaerobic alactate, anaerobic lactate (glycolytic),* and *aerobic.* The energy for short duration, maximal intensity efforts such as throwing the shot put or sprinting 50 meters is generated from the anaerobic alactate system. Anaerobic energy production, so named because it is possible in the absence of oxygen, may be further classified into two categories: the anaerobic alactate (or ATP-PC system, in which creatine phosphate is used in the conversion of ADP to ATP) and the anaerobic lactate (glycolytic) system. The anaerobic alactate system is responsible for fueling events lasting from one to five seconds with an immediate supply of ATP. For intense events lasting more than six seconds there is a gradual shift toward ATP production from the anaerobic lactate or glycolytic system. During events lasting longer than 45 seconds, both anaerobic and aerobic energy systems are needed in combination. As event duration increases, progressively more energy comes from aerobic metabolism. The energy required to perform steady-state exercise lasting greater than 10 minutes results primarily from aerobic metabolism.

We describe distinct natures of these three energy production pathways in order to make them easier to comprehend as well as to convey their unique contributions to overall function. However, in most endurance events there is an interaction of all three pathways.

In many events, such as trials of specified distance or time, the energy demand is relatively balanced, whereas in other events, such as a mountainous bike race or Nordic ski course, the energy demand is highly variable.

During intense exercise that involves the anaerobic lactate or glycolytic system, lactic acid production is increased and pH levels decline. This shift in acidity is compensated in part by regulatory systems including increased ventilation (breathing), buffering systems (bicarbonate system), and renal (kidney) regulation of metabolites. For our purposes, the high-intensity type of interval training that involves anaerobic lactate or the so-called glycolytic pathway (using CHO as a primary fuel source) reduces pH and appears to be responsible for calcium loss. A heightened level of metabolic acidity should not be regarded as an entirely negative consequence of exercise, however, as acidosis may be a necessary precursor for the development of favorable adaptations including increases in specific enzymes that catalyze reactions involving the metabolism of glucose. However, exercise induced acidosis should be considered by endurance athletes as a potential risk factor for loss of bone mass (Krieger, et al., 1992).

In order to maximize training effectiveness and minimize the likelihood of bone loss, the endurance athlete must fully understand the role of exercise intensity and duration as well as the role of interval training as it relates to perturbations in pH. To illustrate the interactions of exercise duration and intensity we highlight the classic work of Sweden's Dr. Per-Olof Astrand. Dr. Astrand is considered one of the fathers of exercise physiology and has researched and published extensively in the areas of physical performance, oxygen transport, and aerobic power. His *Textbook of Work Physiology* (2003) is considered a classic by modern students of exercise science.

A subject whose maximal oxygen consumption was 4.6 L/min was asked to exercise as long as possible at an intensity of 350 W on a cycle ergometer (see Table 8.1). This person was able to sustain this effort level for only eight minutes at which time he was totally exhausted. The amount of oxygen the subject utilized during this test was recorded at 5.2 L/min and therefore recruited anaerobic as well as aerobic energy system participation (5.2 L/min–4.6 L/min = contribution of anaerobic energy production). Both heart rate and lactate levels were maximal (190 bpm, 16 mM). In the next exercise trial, the work rate was decreased by 50% (175 W) and in this case, the subject could exercise easily for 60 minutes with no appreciable rise in blood lactate. Heart rate remained stable at 135 beats per minute while oxygen uptake was consistently 2.45 L/min.

Table 8.1 Summary of continuous exercise

Workload (watts)	Duration (minutes)	Heart rate (beats/min)	VO2 (l/min)	Blood lactate (mM)
350	8	190	4.6	16.5
175	60	135	2.45	1.3

Source: Astrand, et al., 1960, 2003; Essen, 1978.

In a follow up experiment, the same subject exercised at a workload of 350 W but this time the exercise session was divided into work and rest intervals of equal duration. Exercise and rest intervals were set at 30 seconds, one minute, two minutes, and three minutes (see Table 8.2). In all of these interval trials, the subject was capable of achieving the desired amount of work within the 60-minute session. However, the physiological responses were significantly different and depended upon the length of the exercise intervals. When the exercise and rest intervals were set at three minutes each, the subject could proceed only with great difficulty. The oxygen uptake and heart rate were now maximal, as was the peak blood lactate concentration. As the exercise interval was shortened, the subject could perform the desired amount of work with significantly less physiologic stress and reduction in pH.

As you can appreciate, the reason interval training often is chosen by coaches and athletes over continuous or steady-state training methods is that it allows for a greater total amount of work at an elevated intensity level. In understanding the basic exercise physiology as detailed in the above experiments, you can appreciate how training intensity and duration of training may be tailored in order to modulate pH. If exercise intensity is increased for short periods (less than one minute), large increases in acidosis are not achieved. Additionally, maximal recruitment of force production on muscles

Table 8.2 Summary of interval data

Interval length (minutes)	Heart rate (beats/min)	VO2 (l/Min)	Blood lactate (mM)
0.5	150	2.9	2.2
1	167	2.93	5.0
2	178	4.4	10.5
3	188	4.6	13.2

Source: Astrand, et al., 1960, 2003; Essen, 1978.

and bones is realized while fatigue is minimized. As the duration of a work interval is increased beyond one minute, lactate levels rise and pH decreases.

These results are not intended to imply that exercise intervals should always be kept at durations of less than one minute, but rather to enable you to understand more fully what is happening to pH levels as a result of exercise intervals of different lengths. Here is the important point: To stimulate development of the anaerobic energy system (as well as increase aerobic capacity) without creating an overly acidic environment, only relatively short duration, high intensity exercise intervals are necessary. For most athletes, high intensity, short duration interval training sessions bring about significant and rapid improvements in certain fitness parameters relative to the time investment.

In 2006 Gibala and colleagues compared brief, intense training (SIT, Sprint Interval Training) to a more traditional program of high volume, low intensity endurance exercise (ET, Endurance Training). Despite the fact that the total energy expenditure was markedly different between groups (630 kJ for the sprint group versus 6500 kJ for the low intensity group), the performance improvements were similar. In addition, improvements in key aerobic enzymes and increases in muscle glycogen were increased with high-intensity training (see also Burgomaster, et al., 2005). For an excellent review on the topic of interval training, see the literature review by Saunders, et al., 2004, who detail the results of interval training studies published through 2004. Their overview categorizes training studies of endurance athletes working in three ranges of intensity (supramaximal, maximal, and submaximal) relative to VO2 max.

Although certain aspects of conditioning and/or race performance may be attained only through prolonged, high-intensity intervals, endurance athletes and coaches should realize that the risk for bone loss may be increased. Furthermore, the fitness that is gained through prolonged intervals of high intensity appears to be achieved within a short number of training sessions.

Several researchers (Lindsey et al., 1996; Westgarth-Taylor et al., 1997) have studied the effects of high-intensity interval training in cyclists. All athletes in their studies had VO2 max values of greater than 65 ml/min/kg and peak sustained power outputs of approximately 400 W. After baseline testing, the cyclists replaced approximately 15% of their 300 km/week endurance riding with six to 12 sessions of high intensity training. Specifically, the sessions were performed once or twice per week for six weeks and consisted of six to nine work intervals lasting five minutes at approximately 86% VO2 max with one minute rest intervals. Examining these study results, Hawley (1997) concluded that the 4–5% improvements that were realized in peak work rates were achieved after four to six training sessions and that significant improvements were not noted between sessions six through twelve.

The famous New Zealand runner and coach Arthur Lydiard provides this perspective on anaerobic training:

> Athletes who continue to train anaerobically throughout the year, constantly creating large oxygen debts with the resultant accumulation of lactic acid and other waste products, can lower the blood's pH to undesirable levels. The continued low blood pH can upset the nutritive system, by destroying and neutralizing the effects of food vitamins, hence retarding general development; as vitamins do not function well in low blood pH, this meaning that an athlete in this physical state will continually derive little nourishment from his food. The low blood pH can also interfere with the functions of the enzymes, resulting in poorer recovery from training and so making successive training sessions more difficult; upset the nervous system causing the athlete to become disinterested and irritable, this state sometimes being called staleness, another effect of this being that sleep and general concentration is upset and also increases the possibilities of neuromuscular breakdowns.

Flawless technique is critically important for this type of training. You should begin high-intensity intervals only after developing satisfactory technical competence lower-intensity workloads. In addition, it is very important that concentration and focus on technique is never lost at the expense of intensity. This point is particularly true for sports in which injury risk related to poor technique is high, including running and rowing. We often see novice or less talented athletes attempt to improve fitness through sheer effort using in misdirected or dysfunctional movement patterns. Trainers or coaches must be vigilant in maintaining close supervision of athletes who are prone to this behavior. The self-coached athlete should consider that these high intensity efforts are only worthwhile if they are performed in a manner that will facilitate long-term technical excellence in one's chosen sport.

In summary, we would recommend that endurance athletes interested in minimizing the likelihood of bone loss due to exercise-induced acidosis consider building their training programs around two basic types of training. The first is lower-intensity endurance training with a focus on cultivating technique and developing the basic aerobic and metabolic systems. The second is short-duration, higher-intensity intervals to develop the anaerobic metabolic pathways. For most athletes, combining these two types of training will result in significant overall development with minimal risk of bone loss related to perturbations in pH.

It is interesting to note that many legendary endurance athletes have first demonstrated success at the track (or shorter endurance events) before moving to the marathon or other long-distance endurance events. Wes Santee, one of America's greatest milers, ran at the University of Kansas for Coach Bill Easton, who believed "that if a distance man had a good quarter mile-mile time, he could run any event" (Bascomb, 2004, p. 102). Wes, like many quality distance runners, was capable of performing a quarter-mile in less than 60 seconds. Therefore, it appears reasonable that even long-distance endurance specialists may benefit from the performance of intervals or "speed training" sessions that last less than 60 seconds with minimal risk of perturbations in pH.

Those athletes who follow a program of periodized training should realize that the performance improvements that result from high intensity (85–95% VO2 max, training intervals lasting longer than two minutes) are realized relatively quickly. For endurance athletes who do not follow a system of periodization, these types of intervals should be used prudently throughout the year.

An example of a program that utilizes interval training in a methodical way is the "Wolverine Plan" developed by Mike Caviston. Mike is the indoor rowing world record holder in the 40–49 lightweight division as well as a kinesiologist, coach, and now Director of Fitness at the Naval Special Warfare Center in Coronado, California. Mike describes the program design as a pyramid consisting of four different types of workouts, Level 1–4 (he knows that the names lack imagination!). The apex consists of Level 1 workouts and the base of Level 4 workouts. The purpose of Levels 2–4 is to support the Level 1 sessions. The Level 1 workouts are considered the backbone of the training program. They are very demanding and are performed at 95–105% of competition 2K pace. Workouts are scheduled once per week (and every two weeks in September and October). Level 1 workouts make up approximately 3–4% of the total weekly rowing volume. The typical Level 1 workout is 8 X 500 meters, but other variations include 4 X 1000 meters or a 4000 meter pyramid (250m/500m/750m/1000m/750m/500m/250m). A complete description of The Wolverine Plan, named after the University of Michigan mascot, is available at the Concept 2 web site (http://www.concept2.com/forums/wolverineplan.htm).

We encourage endurance athletes to understand fully the nature and intent of interval and high-intensity training. Joe Friel, athlete and respected cycling and triathlon coach, may have described the situation seen in the clinic all too frequently: "In training both elite and recreational athletes, I've noticed a curious difference. Elite riders generally treat high-intensity training as if it's a powerful drug. They use it in carefully measured doses at pre-selected times. Recreational cyclists, on the other hand, almost always devour high intensity as though it's candy." Coach Friel has written many excellent books and has a useful web site (www.joefrielsblog.com).

To quantify and progress interval workouts, we suggest the graphical model developed by Guy Thibault, PhD. Dr. Thibault is an exercise physiologist, a full-time research advisor to the Sport and Leisure Secretariat of the Government of Quebec, and a scientific advisor to the national training centers for several sports in Canada. He is the former coach of Jacqueline Gareau, 1980 winner of the Boston Marathon. With his kind permission, we provide his model here for your personal use.

Thibault's graph is designed to assist coaches and athletes in developing interval training sessions in which duration, intensity, and recovery are well defined. Most endurance athletes can use the graph, which is not sport specific. The model contains six curves that correspond to relative intensity zones of 85–110% of maximal aerobic power. Duration of each work interval is represented on the x-axis, and the number of repetitions on the y-axis. Each point on the curves of the graph represents an interval training session. The squares represent sessions in which work intervals are multiples of 30 seconds. The box in the upper right hand corner provides the duration of active recovery between work intervals and sets. It is assumed that active recovery is low intensity, approximately 50% of maximal aerobic power. The sessions can be made less challenging by reducing the number of repetitions and/or sets. For example, completing five, six, or seven work intervals that could be performed according to the model corresponds to a 50, 60, or 70% difficulty, respectively.

In our experience, as well as that of Dr. Thibault, well-trained athletes are able to adjust their level of effort simply by knowing the pattern of the workout. Specifically, if athletes are instructed in the number of work intervals and the duration of the recovery periods, they should be capable of self-selecting the appropriate pace. For additional information regarding Dr. Thibault's training model please refer to Enhanced Fitness and Performance at http://www.enhancedfp.com.

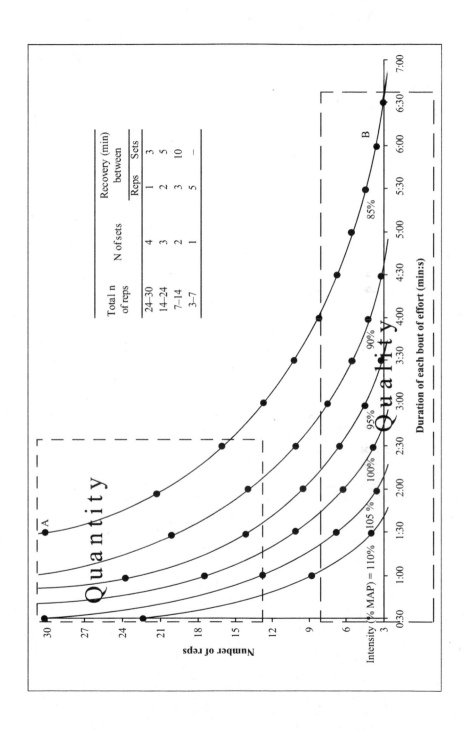

Total n of reps	N of sets	Recovery (min) between	
		Reps	Sets
24–30	4	1	3
14–24	3	2	5
7–14	2	3	10
3–7	1	5	–

Acid-Base Regulation by Dietary Means

Although exercise has the most profound influence on the body's pH, diet can alter calcium flux and bone health through changes in acid-base balance. Classic studies on effects of dietary protein were performed by Hellen Linkswiler and her colleagues (Walker and Linksweiler, 1972; Hegsted and Linkswiler, 1981; Linkswiler, et al., 1981; Zemel, et al., 1981). These studies showed that when excessive protein was added to the diet in the form of purified supplements, calcium balance became negative, suggesting a net loss of bone. Paradoxically, however, when increased protein content from whole food was added to the diets of healthy people, reductions in calcium balance were not always observed. This improved outcome presumably was related to other constituents in whole food, namely phosphate, sulfate, potassium, and calcium. In general, the digestion of meats and some types of grain appears to induce a significant acid load, while fruits and vegetables metabolize in a manner that favors a more basic (alkaline) result. Therefore, the net acid load of high animal protein and grain-based diets, versus the alkaline load of plant-based diets, have been described as factors in systemic calcium balance.

A quotation from Clarence DeMar (1998), winner of seven Boston Marathons and a 1924 Olympic Medal, provides a glimpse of when select athletes first became aware of this strategy:

> The year 1934, notwithstanding in my sixteenth in the B.A.A. developed into a good year for marathoning. I had begun to experiment with some radical ideas of Hauser, Jackson, Bragg and others about diet. Their chief emphasis was to have an alkaline reaction in seventy-five percent of the food. This is found in fresh fruits and vegetables as contrasted to the acid of starches and meats.

Researchers Remer and Manz (1995) have calculated the potential renal acid load (PRAL) of 114 frequently consumed foods based upon 100 g servings. Fruits and vegetables have negative values, meaning they reduce acid excretion; milk and yogurt are neutral to slightly positive; and meats, fish, poultry, cheese, and many grain products create significantly positive acid loads (see Table 8.3). In 1997, Lawrence showed that a diet rich in fruits and vegetables and low in sweets and snacks reduced the amount of urinary calcium loss by nearly 25%. Even more recently, Lanham (2008) demonstrated that by increasing fruit and vegetable consumption, calcium excretion was reduced by 30%. For an excellent reference that highlights

Table 8.3 Average potential renal acid loads (PRAL) of certain food groups and foods

Food group	PRAL
Meat and meat products	+ 9.5
Eggs	+ 8.1
Spaghetti products	+ 6.7
Bread	+ 3.5
Milk and non-cheese products	+ 1.0
High protein cheese (> 15 g protein/100 g)	+ 23.6
Vegetables	
Spinach	–14.0
Carrots	–4.9
Celery	–5.2
Fruits	
Raisins	–21.0
Bananas	– 5.5
Apricots	– 4.8

Source: Remer and Manz, 1995.

the value of diet in regulating bone health through acid-base balance we recommend *Building Bone Vitality: A Revolutionary Diet Plan to Prevent Bone Loss and Reverse Osteoporosis* (Lanou and Castleman, 2009).

Although we are aware of no scientific studies to date that evaluate the merits of consuming a highly alkaline meal before or immediately following highly intense or prolonged endurance exercise, our athletes have reported improved rates of recovery and less delayed muscle soreness with this strategy. Specific guidelines for eating before, during, and after exercise will be presented in Chapter 10.

Summary

Based on substrate utilization, time, and intensity, exercise metabolism can be compartmentalized into three unique but interactive pathways. They are the anaerobic alactate, anaerobic lactate (glycolytic), and aerobic energy systems. These three pathways are all operational to a greater or lesser extent in most endurance sports.

Metabolic acidosis increases in response to high-intensity endurance training and racing and results from the blending of both anaerobic and aerobic energy systems that may pose a risk factor for bone loss. It is important that endurance athletes know how exercise intensity and diet influence body pH in order to protect against or reverse bone loss.

Although historically lactic acid has been considered a cause of fatigue, more contemporary research reveals that it augments rather than inhibits exercise performance. The metabolic acidosis that results from high-intensity exercise appears to be related to the increase in hydrogen ion concentration following the degradation of ATP. However, monitoring lactate levels in training and research settings may still provide useful data as lactate levels are correlated with reductions in pH. The so-called lactate threshold exercise intensity level does not appear to be a discrete point but rather a melding of anaerobic and aerobic metabolic pathways.

Endurance athletes may gauge their levels of preparedness or performance throughout the year by utilizing a standard time or distance trial. As fitness increases, there will be less metabolic acidosis at a given work rate. This is known as shifting the lactate curve to the right. Elite endurance athletes have developed the ability to perform at a very high percentage of their VO2 max for prolonged periods and are capable of producing very high levels of lactate for short durations. The development of these two respective capabilities appears to require extensive dedication, cultivation, and focus.

Interval training methods are popular among athletes and coaches because the total amount of high intensity work that can be accomplished is greater than that which can be achieved with steady state training. High intensity intervals of less than one minute enable an athlete to recruit large motor units, thus providing a stimulus for the development of sport-specific strength and power; yet they do not induce severe reductions in pH. Additionally, the performance gains associated with longer duration, high-intensity intervals (anaerobic lactate or glycolytic system) appear to be realized relatively quickly. For the athlete interested in minimizing bone loss related to exercise-induced acidosis, only a minimal amount of training time appears necessary or prudent.

In addition to the increased calcium excretion that is associated with high-intensity endurance exercise, diet also may play an important role in the maintenance of pH. Although the exact mechanisms of how certain foods influence the skeleton has yet to be precisely defined, the so-called acid ash theory (referring to the pH of the residue thought to result from food breakdown) has been in place for many years. Research indicates that certain foods are digested and metabolized in a manner that results in either an acidic or an alkaline state. Foods known to induce the greatest degree of acidosis and corresponding calcium excretion are meats, grains, and hard cheeses. In contrast, a plant-based diet rich in fruits and vegetables is known to reduce calcium loss and improve bone strength, presumably due to the creation of an alkaline environment.

REFERENCES

Astrand I, Astrand PO, Christensen EH, Hedman R (1960) Intermittent muscular work. *Acta Physiologica Scandinavica* 48:448–453.

Astrand PO, Rodahl K, Dahl H, Stromme S (2003) *Textbook of Work Physiology, Physiologic Bases of Exercise*. Fourth Edition. Human Kinetics: Champaign, IL.

Bascomb N (2004) *The Perfect Mile*. New York, NY: Houghton Mifflin Company.

Burgomaster K, Hughes S, Heigenhauser G, Bradwell S, Gibala M (2005) Six sessions of sprint interval training increases muscle oxidative potential and cycle endurance capacity in humans. *Journal of Applied Physiology* 98:1985–1990.

DeMar C (1998) Some victories in my old age, Chapter 13 in *Marathon: The Clarence DeMar Story*. Medway, OH:Cedarwinds Publishing.

Dressendorfer R, Peterson S, Lovshin S, Keen C (2002) Mineral metabolism in male cyclists during high-intensity endurance training. *International Journal of Sport and Exercise Metabolism* 12(1):63–72.

Essen B (1978) Studies on the regulation of metabolism in human skeletal muscle using intermittent exercise as an experimental model. *Acta Physiologica Scandinavica* Suppl., Vol. 454:1–32.

Friel J (1996) *The Cyclist's Training Bible. A Complete Training Guide for the Competitive Road Cyclist*. Boulder, Colorado: VeloPress.

Gibala M, Little J, van Essen M, Wilkin G, Burgomaster K, Safdar A, Raha S, Tarnopolsky M (2006) Short-term sprint interval versus traditional endurance training: similar initial adaptations in human skeletal muscle and exercise performance. *Journal of Physiology* 575:901–911.

Hawley J, Myburgh KH, Noakes T, Dennis SC (1997) Training techniques to improve fatigue resistance and endurance performance. *Journal of Sports Science* 15:325–333.

Hegsted M, Linkswiler HM (1981) Long-term effects of level of protein intake on calcium metabolism in young adult women. *Journal of Nutrition* 111:244–251.

Krieger N, Sessler N, Bushinsky D (1992) Acidosis inhibits osteoblastic and stimulates osteoclastic activity in vitro. *American Journal of Physiology* 262:F442–448.

Lanham S (2008) The balance of bone health: tipping the scales in favor of potassium-rich, bicarbonate-rich foods. *Journal of Nutrition* 138:172S–177S.

Lanou A, Castleman M (2009) *Building Bone Vitality*. New York: McGraw-Hill.

Lindsay F, Hawley J, Myburgh KH, Schomer HH, Noakes TD, Dennis SC (1996) Improved athletic performance in highly trained cyclists after interval training. *Medicine and Science in Sports and Exercise* 28:1427–1434.

Linkswiler HM, Zemel MB, Hegsted M, Schuette S (1981) Protein-induced hypercalciuria. *Federation Proceedings* 40:2429–2433.

Lawrence J (1997) A clinical trial of the effects of dietary patterns on blood pressure. *The New England Journal of Medicine* 336:1117–1124.

Remer T, Manz F (1995) Potential renal acid load of foods and its influence on urine pH. *Journal of the American Dietetic Association* 95:791–797.

Saunders P, Pyne D, Foster C (2004) Effects of high-intensity training on performance and physiology of endurance athletes. Online at sportsci.org 8:25–40.

Sheehan G (1978) *Running and Being*. New York: Simon and Schuster.

Ullyot J(1978) *The Complete Marathoner*. Emmaus, PA:World Publications.

Walker RM, Linkswiler HM (1972) Calcium retention in the adult male is affected by protein intake. *Journal of Nutrition* 102:1297–1302.

Westgarth-Taylor C, Hawley JA, Rickard S, Myburgh KH, Noakes TD, Dennis SC (1997) Metabolic and performance adaptations to interval training in endurance trained cyclists. *European Journal of Applied Physiology* 75:298–304.

Zemel MB, Schuette S, Hegsted M, Linkswiler HM (1981) Role of the sulfur-containing amino acids in protein-induced hypercalciuria in men. *Journal of Nutrition* 111:545–552.

CHAPTER NINE

Calcium

Calcium is the most common mineral in the human body. The majority of this element is stored in the skeleton, where it exists mainly in the form of hydroxyapatite crystals containing large amounts of both calcium and phosphate. Beyond its structural importance, calcium functions in the body to maintain blood pressure, nerve transmission, muscle contraction, glycogen mobilization, and hormone regulation. Calcium is so critical to our survival for all of these biochemical and physiological needs that if dietary intake is inadequate, the skeleton will be demineralized in a sacrifice of structural integrity to functional imperatives. Because endurance athletes place such heavy demands on their systems during training and competition, their intake of calcium is particularly critical so that skeletal health will not be sacrificed to peak athletic performance. We stress strongly here that bone mass should not be considered as a static structural framework of the body, but as fully dynamic a functional physiological element as muscle mechanics, blood pressure fluctuations, and nerve transmission.

Because of its biological significance, calcium levels in the body are tightly controlled by several interrelated mechanisms. Key components include parathyroid hormone (PTH), vitamin D, and calcitonin. PTH is released by the parathyroid glands, located in the neck, in response to low levels of blood calcium. PTH causes the gastrointestinal tract to increase calcium absorption from food, acts directly on bone by increasing resorption through an osteoblast-RANKL mediated pathway, and causes the kidneys to excrete more phosphorous, which indirectly raises calcium levels. Although this highly integrated system allows for responsive and tight control of blood calcium levels, it does so at the potential expense of the skeleton.

Vitamin D works collaboratively with PTH on the bones and kidneys and is required for intestinal calcium absorption. Vitamin D can be obtained through dietary sources or as a product of sun exposure. The hormone calcitonin, released by the thyroid, parathyroid, and thymus glands, decreases blood calcium levels by promoting the incorporation of calcium into bone.

Calcium is absorbed from food in the small intestine and transported in the bloodstream to various body targets by a carrier protein. Bone resorption increases in response to low blood calcium levels. If resorption is prolonged, irreversible bone loss may occur.

Unfortunately, researchers continue to find that calcium remains one of the nutrients most frequently lacking in the diets of endurance specialists. For example, a 1994 study by Estok and Rudy of female runners' diets reported that out of 17 nutrients examined, only calcium levels were inadequate. In another study of Division 1-A athletes by Leachman-Slawson, and colleagues (2001), female crosscountry athletes reported the lowest average calcium intake at only 605 mg/day. More than a decade earlier, Myburgh and co-workers (1990) had reported that stress fractures were 12 times more frequent in people with low dietary calcium intakes and low calcium intake was by far the best predictor for risk of stress fracture.

Daily calcium requirements can be achieved by eating a combination of calcium-rich foods, calcium-fortified foods, and/or supplemental calcium sources. Most health professionals recommend that foods naturally high in calcium should be the first choice in meeting daily calcium requirements. Whole foods that contain calcium provide many other essential nutrients as well as other health-promoting ingredients that are absent in calcium supplements (Tables 9.1, 9.2).

Table 9.1 Dietary requirements for calcium intake

Age	Calcium DRI (mg/day)
9–18 years	1,300
19–50 years	1,000
51–70 years	1,200
>71 years	1,200

Source: National Academy of Science's Food and Nutrition Board (1997).

Table 9.2 Calcium-rich foods (300 mg)

Food	Serving size
Milk	1 c
Cottage cheese	2 c
Yogurt	1 c
Broccoli	2 c
Collard greens	1 c
Turnip greens	1 c
Mustard greens	1.5 c
Canned salmon with bone	4 oz
Sardines	3 oz
Goat's milk	1 c
Blackstrap molasses	2 tbsp
Sesame seeds	.25 c
Tofu	8–10 oz
Swiss cheese	1.5 oz
Spinach	1 c
Swiss chard	3 c
Kale	3 c

Calcium-fortified Foods

Because of the health concerns about senile osteoporosis and because most people have inadequate calcium intake, food manufacturers have began marketing calcium-fortified foods. The list of fortified foods includes juices, cereals, spreads, and water. Unfortunately, the bioavailability and absorption of calcium from these fortified sources is uncertain (the bioavailability of a nutrient refers to the degree of actual absorption relative to what is consumed). Thus, it is very possible that the calcium content on the product label may be significantly greater than the amount that your body actually assimilates.

Supplemental calcium is available in two basic forms: carbonate and citrate. Calcium carbonate is the most common type and is available in many forms, including capsules, tablets, and chews. Although it is the least expensive to produce, it is absorbed poorly in people with decreased stomach acid (elderly individuals or those on anti-acid medications). Also, because it requires stomach acid to be digested and absorbed, calcium carbonate supplements must be taken at mealtime.

Calcium citrate is more expensive to produce but is better absorbed and is less likely to cause bloating than calcium carbonate. Some researchers suggest that this form of calcium may protect against the development of kidney stones. Because it contains acid it may be taken without food.

Because calcium absorption in the body is limited to about 500 mg per dose, we recommend spreading your calcium intake throughout the day. As we will discuss in further detail in Chapter 10, you should include a calcium-rich food source or supplement in your pre-exercise meal. Additionally, we encourage you to consider a midnight snack that contains calcium. Although the literature is not consistent regarding the value of consuming a nighttime calcium supplement, the balance of support appears to favor this tactic as being effective in suppressing the nocturnal rise in bone resorption activity. In 1994 Blumsohn and colleagues administered 1,000 mg of elemental calcium in the form of calcium citrate for 14 days at either 08:00 or 23:00 hours to nine subjects. Samples of blood and urine were collected and biochemical markers of bone cell activity were evaluated. The group that received the evening dose of supplemental calcium demonstrated a significant suppression of two markers of bone resorption (deoxypyridinoline and N-telopeptide of type I collagen). In 2008 another group of researchers (Adolphi, et al.) studied the effects of bedtime consumption of a fermented milk product on bone cell activity by measuring biochemical markers of bone formation and resorption. The results demonstrated that the fermented milk product also reduced the nocturnal excretion of deoxypyridinoline.

Even in the case of natural foods, the bioavailability of calcium can be influenced by several factors that you should consider when planning this aspect of your diet. Certain foods, including calcium-rich, dark-green leafy vegetables, contain substances called *oxalates.* Oxalates, or oxalic acid, may bind with calcium and reduce its absorption. However, it is possible to improve the calcium availability in these foods by boiling them in water for a few seconds. A decrease of 5–15% of oxalate content can be achieved with this blanching (quick boiling) technique. Other foods that contain oxalates that may compromise calcium absorption include:

- Black tea
- Chocolate
- Nuts (almonds, cashews)

- Wheat bran
- Soybeans and soy products
- Blackberries
- Blueberries
- Kiwi fruit

We do not recommend eliminating foods containing oxalates from your diet, since many are actually good calcium sources themselves. However, it is important to remember that when you eat foods that contain oxalates, total calcium utilization is less than the total calcium you actually consumed. Other factors can reduce the bioavailability of calcium as well.

Fiber

Fiber is a non-starch polysaccharide that makes up much of the structure of leaves, stems, seeds, and fruit and vegetable skins. Although fiber is increasingly recognized as an important component of a healthy diet, excessive fiber intake can decrease the absorption of dietary minerals, including calcium. The current recommendation for fiber consumption is 20–35 g per day (see Table 9.3).

Table 9.3 Fiber content of selected foods

Food	Serving size	Fiber (g)
Oatmeal	1 c	4
Green lentils	¼ c dry	9
All bran cereal	1 c	17
Pinto beans	1 c cooked	20
Pumpkin seeds	1 oz	10
Peanuts	1 oz	3.5
Walnuts	1 oz	1.6
Pear	1	5
Blueberries	1 c	4

Caffeine

Caffeine is a diuretic, which causes an obligatory increase in calcium loss through urine excretion. Caffeine intake below 400 mg per day (the amount in two to four cups of coffee) should not have a significant effect on calcium status.

Sodium

Excessive salt intake also increases urinary excretion of calcium. The current recommendation for sodium intake is 2,400 mg per day—but the average American consumes two to three times this amount! A longitudinal study of 40 postmenopausal females found that limiting sodium intake (2,000 mg/day) for six months produced significant reductions in calcium excretion and aminoterminal propeptide of type I collagen, a marker of bone resorption (Carbone, et al., 2005). An athletes' sodium intakes are highly variable and dependent upon a variety of factors including habitual intake, fitness, and environmental acclimatization. In general, as an athlete consumes less salt, becomes more fit, and trains in the heat, the body's sodium conservation mechanisms improve and thus sodium requirements are decreased.

Protein

Foods that cause reductions in pH, including many sources of protein, can increase calcium excretion. The influence of protein consumption on calcium balance is part of a complex interplay among several factors, including the overall dietary pH, total protein intake, protein source, and the calcium-to-protein ratio.

Calcium Toxicity

Toxicity from dietary calcium overload is rare because excessive calcium intake is countered by a reduction in gastrointestinal tract absorption. However, constipation and an increased risk of kidney stones have been reported. Excessive calcium levels are more likely to be related to hormonal abnormalities and/or to be a consequence of certain cancers. Symptoms of hypercalcemia include:

- Nausea and vomiting
- Constipation
- Abdominal pain
- Muscle weakness

There are few reports of toxicity from calcium ingestion, but chronic calcium overload may result in an excessively alkaline stomach, which makes it difficult to digest certain foods difficult (milk-alkali syndrome). Additionally, since there is competitive absorption between calcium and other minerals (zinc, iron, magnesium) in the small intestine, it is also possible that a high calcium intake may limit the absorption of other minerals.

Currently, the recommended safe upper limit for daily calcium intake is set at 2,500 mg and there is no significant evidence that more is better for general maintenance. However, both cardiac and skeletal muscle contractions are calcium dependent, and calcium losses in perspiration may be significant. Thus, in certain circumstances, endurance athletes may require a higher amount than what is traditionally recommended.

Barry and colleagues (2008) studied changes in bone mineral density values over one year of training and competition in 14 competitive male cyclists. Subjects were randomized to receive either 1,500 mg (500 mg with each meal) or 250 mg of supplemental calcium citrate daily. Bone mineral density decreased significantly during the season, with no difference found between the two levels of calcium supplementation. The two-hour dermal calcium loss was estimated at 136.5 +/− 60.5 mg. It is not known whether higher levels of calcium supplementation would have reduced bone loss in these athletes. Dr. Eric Orwoll, Director of the Oregon Health and Science University in Portland and an authority on male osteoporosis, said in a 2004 interview for *Bicycling Magazine*, "You can speculate all you want about cycling and osteoporosis, but get enough calcium and vitamin D and you're okay" (Wallack, 2004).

Training Influences on Calcium Requirements

Calcium requirements for athletes may vary during the year and be dependent upon such factors as the athlete's size, training volume (and intensity), environmental conditions, overall diet quality, protein intake, and the maintenance of energy balance.

During an "off season" in which an athlete is participating in only minimal or moderate levels of formal training and engaging in recreational pursuits (hiking, walking, yoga, flexibility/mobility exercise, sub-maximal strength training) of less than or equal to two hours/day, calcium requirement (along with total energy and protein intake) will be relatively low: Calcium requirement: 1,200–2,400 mg/day. For people with normal bone mass and minimal activity, the lower end of the calcium range may be sufficient. Individuals who have been diagnosed with low bone mass or who have higher levels of energy expenditure should aim for the upper end of the range.

When an athlete is engaged in heavy training, total dietary energy intake, protein, and calcium requirements will be significantly greater: Calcium requirement: 1,500–3,000 mg/day. The lower end of the daily calcium range may be acceptable for those with normal bone mass and lower volume training days. The upper end of the range may be recommended for those who have been diagnosed with low bone mass or have higher levels of energy expenditure.

Because calcium is metabolized during exercise at an accelerated rate and also is lost in perspiration, calcium requirements may be significantly increased during training or racing in environments with high ambient temperatures. For example, an athlete who runs a marathon (26.2 miles) that requires four hours to complete, or rides in a bicycle century (100 miles) lasting six hours, may lose 400–1,200 mg of calcium in sweat alone.

We recommend taking supplemental calcium at a rate of 100–200 mg per hour of exercise. If your sports drink does not contain calcium, calcium tablets can be easily crushed and dissolved in a commercial sports drink.

In a landmark study published by Lappe and colleagues (2008), over 5,000 female U.S. Navy recruits were divided randomly into two groups. Half of the women in this double-blind study were given 2,000 mg of supplemental calcium and 800 IU of vitamin D; the other half was given a placebo. Among the 3,700 recruits who completed the study, a 21% lower incidence of stress fractures was observed in the supplemented versus control group (6.8% versus 8.6%).

Vitamin D

In order to maximize calcium's effectiveness on the skeleton as well as garner many other health benefits, adequate vitamin D must be consumed. Vitamin D is a group of fat-soluble prohormones with various forms; the two major types are D2 (ergocalciferol) and D3 (cholecalciferol). Vitamin D regulates calcium levels in the blood by promoting absorption in the intestine and re-absorption in the kidneys. It also may act indirectly on bone through the development of stronger muscle contractions.

In addition to having a powerful influence on the musculoskeletal system, adequate vitamin D intake has been recognized as being important in the prevention of cancer, coronary disease, hypertension, and diabetes. Unfortunately, we suspect that many endurance athletes have chronically low vitamin D levels, which may increase their susceptibility to these disease processes as well as to osteoporosis and stress fractures.

Some objective scientific studies provide data in support of these suspicions of dietary shortcomings in endurance athletes. For example, Nieman and colleagues (1989) evaluated three-day diet recall of a large group of male and female marathon runners (291 men, 56 women) and compared these records to various standards of dietary quality. Intake by the runners exceeded two-thirds of the recommended dietary allowance for all nutrients except vitamin D and zinc in females. Even more critically, the research institute of military medicine in Helsinki, Finland, has reported that a lower level of vitamin D is a predisposing element for bone stress fractures (Ruohola, et al., 2006) (see Table 9.4).

Table 9.4 Current recommendation for vitamin D

Age (years)	DRI (International Units)
Birth to 50	200
51–70	400
>71	600

Source: National Academy of Sciences.

Vitamin D needs can be met by diet or sun exposure; in the latter case it is produced by a photochemical reaction that occurs primarily in the outer skin layers. A critical determinant of vitamin D production is the presence and concentration of melanin, which absorbs light. Individuals with darker skin (containing more melanin) require more sun exposure to produce the same amount of vitamin D as do individuals with lighter skin. Additionally, both the season of the year and the distance that one resides from the equator influence vitamin D production. People living in snowy regions are likely to produce inadequate vitamin D from sun exposure alone during the winter months.

Young adults can achieve adequate levels of vitamin D if they receive about 10–15 minutes of sun exposure most days of the week. However, such short exposures may not be adequate for people over 50 years, since vitamin D production declines with age. The use of artificial sunscreens also can effectively block the production of vitamin D.

The best food sources of vitamin D are fatty seafood, particularly cold-water fish (see Table 9.5). Very few routinely consumed

Table 9.5 Natural dietary sources of vitamin D

Food	Serving size	Vitamin D (IU)
Cod liver oil	1 tbs	1,360
Herring	3 oz	1,383
Salmon	3 oz	360
Mackerel	3 oz	345
Whole egg	1 large	20

foods contain meaningful amounts of vitamin D. Consequently, manufacturers have fortified certain foods, particularly dairy products. Unfortunately, most of this supplementation adds very little; for example, a typical cup of milk contains only 100 IU of vitamin D. Therefore, to ensure adequate levels of vitamin D, most athletes are likely to need a supplemental regime. We recommend consulting your primary care physician, who can determine your vitamin D levels with a simple blood test. Additionally, because vitamin D levels are affected by age and season (sun exposure), repeated testing is advisable.

New scientific research shows that supplemental doses may be necessary to confer vitamin D's health benefits including reduced fracture risk. In a review of the scientific studies performed to date, Bischoff-Ferrari and colleagues (2009) reported that oral vitamin D supplementation between 700–800 IU per day appears to reduce the risk of hip and any non-vertebral fractures in ambulatory or institutionalized elderly persons. Although the official safe current upper limit is 2,000 IU per day, many researchers (e.g. Vieth, 2004) are encouraging that levels of vitamin D in the 2,000–4,000 IU per day range be prescribed. These higher doses have proven to be safe, and actually may be necessary to increase blood levels to the minimal therapeutic 90–120 nmol/l range. The normal physiologic limit of vitamin D in the blood may extend to as high as 200 nmol/l (80 ng/ml).

A recent article by Willis and colleagues (2008) in the *International Journal of Sports Nutrition and Exercise Metabolism* noted a surprisingly high worldwide prevalence of vitamin D deficiency. Not only is vitamin D necessary for optimal bone health, but emerging evidence suggests that inadequate vitamin D status increases the risk of developing autoimmune and nonskeletal chronic diseases and also can have a profound effect on immunity, inflammation, and muscle function in the elderly. Extrapolating from this general situation, they suggested that although very little is known about vitamin D status among athletes, poor vitamin D status is likely to be a problem among them as well. Compromised vitamin D status can influence an athlete's overall health and ability to train by affecting innate immunity, exercise-related immunity, and inflammation. Although further research in this area is needed, we encourage sports nutritionists to assess vitamin D and calcium intake and make appropriate recommendations that will help athletes achieve adequate vitamin D status, defined as serum 25(OH) D of at least 75 or 80 nmol/L.

In addition to the multitude of health benefits conferred by adequate vitamin D status, endurance athletes who have been vitamin D deficient also may anticipate a reduction in musculoskeletal pain, especially lower back pain, following the restoration of normal vitamin D levels (Bahr, et al., 2004; Hangai, et al., 2009). Although no studies to date have specifically evaluated the relationship between vitamin D status and pain in an athletic population, this correlation has been identified in non-exercising groups. The mechanism by which vitamin D deficiency leads to bone pain is:

Vitamin D deficiency causes a reduction in calcium absorption
⇊
Production of PTH is increased
(to maintain blood calcium levels)
⇊
PTH results in increased urinary excretion of phosphorus
(hypophosphatemia)
⇊
Insufficient calcium phosphate leads to reductions in the mineral content of the collagen matrix of bone
⇊
When collagen matrix hydrates and swells, it causes pressure on the sensory-innervated regions (periosteum) of bone leading to pain

The pain that seems to develop as a result of vitamin D deficiency is described as being dull and achy in nature and fails to improve with pharmaceutical or physical treatments. Pain levels appear to be significantly improved or abolished within 12 weeks of high-dose vitamin D supplementation (4,000–5,000 IU vitamin D/day); see Faraj and Mutairi, (2003) and Schwalfenberg (2009).

Summary

The relationship between calcium intake and bone health is well established. Unfortunately, many endurance athletes consume less calcium than is considered baseline even for the non-exercising population. Because calcium is lost through sweat, is necessary for muscle contraction, and acts as a buffer to offset exercise-induced acidosis, endurance athletes may require more calcium than the amounts generally recommended. Calcium intake should be tailored individually and reflect multiple factors, including body size, energy expenditure, environmental conditions, individual sweating rates, dietary quality, protein intake, and dietary sources of calcium. Additional considerations for calcium intake include certain factors that limit its absorption including competition between other minerals, fiber, oxalates, sodium, and caffeine. Whole food sources of calcium are generally considered better than manufactured supplements because bioavailability is likely to be superior in whole foods.

The incorporation of calcium into bone is contingent on adequate vitamin D levels. Recent evidence reveals that most populations, including athletes, are vitamin D deficient. Whole food sources of vitamin D are uncommon, so we believe that supplemental D is mandatory, especially in cooler climates where sun exposure is limited. Intake and circulating vitamin D levels often are not correlated, so vitamin D levels should be evaluated with a simple blood test. We encourage endurance athletes to closely scrutinize both calcium and vitamin D levels in order to minimize bone loss and maximize general health.

REFERENCES

Adolphi B, Scholz-Ahrens KE, de Vrese M, Açil Y, Laue C, Schrezenmeir J (2008) Short-term effect of bedtime consumption of fermented milk supplemented with calcium, inulin-type fructans, and caseinphosphopeptides on bone metabolism in healthy, postmenopausal women. *European Journal of Nutrition* 48(1):45–53.

Bahr R, Anderson S, Loken S, Fossan B, Hansen T, Holme I (2004) Low back pain among endurance athletes with and without specific back loading-a cross sectional survey of cross-country skiers, rowers, orienteerers, and non-athletic controls. *Spine* 29:449–454.

Barry D, Kohrt W (2008) BMD decreases over the course of a year in competitive male cyclists. *Journal of Bone and Mineral Research* 23(4):484–491.

Bischoff-Ferrari HA, Willett WC, Wong JB, Stuck AE, Staehelin HB, Orav EJ, Thoma A, Kiel DP, Henschkowski J (2009) Prevention of nonvertebral fractures with oral vitamin D and dose dependency: a meta-analysis of randomized controlled trials. *Archives of Internal Medicine* 169(6):551–561.

Blumsohn A, Herrington K, Hannon R, Shao P, Eyre D (1994) The effect of calcium supplementation on the circadian rhythm of bone resorption. *Journal of Clinical Endocrinology and Metabolism* 79(3):730–735.

Carbone L, Barrow K, Bush A (2005) Effects of a low sodium diet on bone metabolism. *Journal of Bone and Mineral Metabolism* 23(6):506–513.

Estok P, Rudy E (1994) Nutrient intake of women runners and nonrunners. *Health Care for Women International* 15(5):435–451.

Faraj A, Mutairi K (2003) Vitamin D deficiency and chronic low back pain in Saudi Arabia. *Spine* 28:177–179.

Hangai M, Kaneoka K, Hinotsu S, Shimizu K, Okubo Y, Miyakawa S, Mukai N, Sakane M, Ochiai N (2009) Lumbar intervertebral disk degeneration in athletes. *American Journal of Sports Medicine* 37(1):149–155.

Lappe J, Cullen D, Haynatski G, Recker R, Ahlf R, Thompson K (2008) Calcium and vitamin D supplementation decreases incidence of stress fractures in female navy recruits. *Journal of Bone and Mineral Research* 23(5):741–749.

Leachman-Slawson D, McClanahan BS, Clemens LH, Ward KD, Klesges RC, Vukadinovich CM, Cantler ED (2001) Food sources of calcium in a sample of African-American and Euro-American collegiate athletes. *International Journal of Sports Nutrition and Exercise Metabolism* 11(2):199–208.

Myburgh K, Hutchins J, Fataar A, Hough S, Noakes T (1990) Low bone density is an etiologic factor for stress fractures in athletes. *Annals of Internal Medicine* 113: 754–759.

Nieman D, Butler J, Pollett L, Dietrich S, Lutz R (1989) Nutrient intake of marathon runners. *Journal of the American Dietetic Association* 89(9): 1273–1278.

Ruohola J, Laaksi I, Ylikomi T, Haataja R, Mattila V, Sahi T, Tuohimaa P, Pihlajamaki H (2006) Association between serum 25(OH)D concentrations and bone stress fractures in Finnish young men. *Journal of Bone and Mineral Research* 21(9):1483–1488.

Schwalfenberg G (2009) Improvement of chronic back pain of failed back surgery with vitamin D repletion: a case series. *The Journal of the American Board of Family Medicine* 22(1):69–74.

Vieth R (2004) Why the optimal requirement for vitamin D3 is probably much higher than what is officially recommended for adults. *Journal of Steroid Biochemistry and Molecular Biology* 89–90(1–5):575–579.

Wallack R (2004) Special Medical Report, Why You Need to Bone Up. *Bicycling Magazine*, March, 50–54.

Willis K, Peterson N, Larson-Meyer D (2008) Should we be concerned about the vitamin D status of athletes? *International Journal of Sports Nutrition and Exercise Metabolism* 18(2):204–224.

CHAPTER TEN

Nutrient Timing

It is already clear that what you eat has a significant effect on overall health, skeletal health, and endurance performance. But recent scientific research is beginning to show that *when* you eat is also important. This chapter provides some guidelines for feeding before, during, and after exercise in order to maximize performance and recovery while minimizing bone loss.

Scientific studies on feeding endurance athletes prior to exercise have used a variety of different methods, and as a result, comparing the studies precisely is difficult. Some studies have had athletes follow meal plans in which either the amount of food (over fed or under fed) or composition of the diet (more carbohydrate or lower carbohydrate) is different from habitual consumption. Many of these studies did not allow adequate time for adaptation to occur. With those caveats, the sports nutrition research indicates that endurance performance may be improved if an athlete: (1) engages in a carbohydrate-loading protocol for three to seven days; (2) eats a carbohydrate-rich meal approximately three hours prior to competition; and/or (3) utilizes supplemental carbohydrates (sports drinks or energy gels) during exercise. Each of these strategies appears to be equally effective at increasing liver glycogen and/or maintaining elevated blood glucose levels for a given exercise session.

This advice is based on controlled scientific research. In 1991 Wright and colleagues examined the effects of no carbohydrate (PP), pre-exercise carbohydrate meal (CP), carbohydrate feedings during exercise (PC), and the combination of carbohydrate feedings before and during exercise (CC) on the metabolic responses during exercise and on exercise performance. Nine trained male cyclists exercised at 70% of maximal intensity until exhaustion. When carbohydrates were consumed, the rate of carbohydrate oxidation was significantly higher throughout exercise than PP. Total work produced during exercise was 19–46% higher when carbohydrates were consumed. Time to exhaustion was 44% (CC), 32% (PC), and 18% (CP) greater than PP. Performance was improved by ingestion of carbohydrates before and/or during exercise; performance was further improved by their combination.

Athletes may incorporate all three practices to a greater or lesser extent, depending upon personal preference, starting times, and the availability of supplements during competition. For example, if an athlete's habitual diet is moderate in carbohydrate and fat intake, a switch to a slightly higher carbohydrate intake for three days, in addition to a carbohydrate rich breakfast, may be helpful for a high intensity cycling time trial race, during which there is no time to be lost for fueling during the race. In contrast, the maintenance of an athlete's standard diet (moderate carbohydrate and fat intake) for the days leading to an ultra distance event may be reasonable provided the race course is well stocked with supplemental carbohydrate and the athlete has the opportunity to consume a pre-race meal containing adequate carbohydrate.

Eating Before Exercise

In the interest of performance enhancement, many investigators have evaluated the role of the pre-exercise meal. Specific attention has been paid to the glycemic index (GI).

The glycemic index provides an approximately quantified value for an ingested carbohydrate's ability to raise blood glucose levels. Blood sugar increase, called the glycemic response, is determined after ingesting a food containing 50 g of a carbohydrate and comparing it over a two-hour period to a standard for carbohydrate (glucose), which has an assigned value of 100. Responses by different individuals range from high to low and can be represented as a frequency distribution in the form of a normal curve. The GI expresses the percentage of total area under the curve for blood glucose response for a specific food compared to glucose. Foods that have a GI of greater than 60 are considered high; those with a GI of less than 40 are considered low. For a complete food list with corresponding GI values, we suggest the following web site: www.glycemicindex. com.

In addition to the short list in Table 10.1, Foster-Powell, et al. (2002) provide a table of glycemic index and glycemic load values for

Table 10.1 Glycemic index levels of some common foods

High GI	Moderate GI	Low GI
White rice	Oatmeal	Lentils
White bread	Pasta	grapefruit
Glucose	Corn	Apples
Cooked carrots	Oranges	Kidney beans
Honey	Peas	Peanuts
Glucose	Sucrose	Fructose
Gatorade	Cytomax	PR-Bar, Ironman
Grapenuts	Powerade	Skim or low fat milk
Cheerios	Cream of wheat	Barley

a wide variety of foods, and Gretebeck, et al. (2002) give a list of popular sports drinks and energy foods.

It long has been believed that athletes who consume high-GI carbohydrates shortly before exercise may experience premature fatigue. The reasoning is that when a high-GI food is consumed, the pancreas releases insulin, a hormone that facilitates the transport of circulating glucose into storage (muscle and adipose tissue). Sharp spikes in insulin lead to significant reductions in blood glucose levels. This condition is known as reactive or rebound hypoglycemia, as blood glucose concentrations may even drop below fasting levels. In addition, high insulin levels increase systemic inflammatory pathways and limit the mobilization and availability of free fatty acids for energy production.

These unfavorable metabolic consequences appear to be reduced by consuming high-GI carbohydrates well in advance of exercise (> 2+ hours) to enable time for insulin and blood glucose levels to return to baseline and/or by consuming carbohydrates that have a lower GI closer to the start of exercise.

In 2001 Kirwan and colleagues performed a study at our facility, The Pennsylvania State University, comparing breakfast cereals with either moderate or high GI carbohydrate. Six males were fed 75 g of carbohydrate in the form of two different cereals, rolled oats (moderate GI, 61) or puffed rice (high GI, 82), combined with 300 ml of water. A control group had water alone. The trials were randomized and the meals were eaten 45 minutes before the subjects performed cycling exercise (60% VO2 peak) to exhaustion. Before exercise, both test meals elicited significant hyperglycemia and hyperinsulinemia compared with control. During exercise, plasma glucose levels were higher at 60 and 90 minutes after the moderate GI meal than they were after either the high GI or the control. Total carbohydrate oxidation was greater during the moderate GI trial than in the control and was directly correlated with exercise performance time. Exercise time was prolonged after the moderate GI trial compared to control, but the high GI trial was not different from the control (moderate 165 + / – 11, high 141 + / – 8, control 134 + / – 13 minutes). The study concluded that, when consumed 45 minutes before exercise, a moderate GI meal provides a significant performance and metabolic advantage.

The results reported by Kirwan and his colleagues accord with numerous previous studies that have shown that a low GI meal consumed prior to competition may improve performance relative to a high GI meal by delaying fatigue. Several investigators have reported that low-glycemic index, pre-exercise feedings were accompanied by higher blood glucose levels near the end stages of exercise (Thomas, et al., 1991, 1994; Burke, et al., 1993; Guezennec, et al., 1993).

The ideal pre-exercise meal should be a source of carbohydrate sufficient to maintain blood glucose and muscle metabolism with minimal perturbations of insulin. A relatively baseline level of insulin should maintain blood glucose availability, optimize fat mobilization, and spare glycogen reserves. Additionally, a low GI pre-exercise meal may provide additional benefits to the skeleton, as demonstrated recently by Chen and colleagues (2009) from the Chinese University of Hong Kong. These investigators evaluated eight trained male runners after they consumed either a high-GI (83) or low-GI (36) meal prior to a 21-km treadmill run. During the experiment, subjects also were provided with supplemental carbohydrate beverages. No differences were found in time to complete the 21-km run between high and low GI trials. However, cortisol concentrations were found to be significantly lower during the low GI condition. Cortisol is a stress hormone that is known to have catabolic effects on bone.

In addition to starting exercise with energy stores at or near full capacity, athletes should strive for optimal hydration status in order to minimize the catabolic consequences of exercise. For example, Maresh and colleagues (2006) evaluated nine male collegiate runners in states of normal hydration and 5% hypohydration. They studied both testosterone and cortisol while the runners exercised at 70% and 85% VO2 max. The researchers found that during the hypohydrated trial, cortisol concentrations were significantly elevated during exercise and remained so for 20 minutes following exercise. Testosterone levels were not altered, but the testosterone-to-cortisol ratio during the 70% trial was significantly lower 20 minutes post-exercise. These findings suggest that hydration status prior to starting exercise can influence the balance between anabolism and catabolism.

We recommend a pre-exercise meal that includes a calcium-rich food source (fortified or naturally occurring) or approximately 300–500 mg of supplemental calcium with vitamin D. In 2004, Guillemant . and colleagues evaluated 12 elite male triathletes in the age range of 23–37 years during 60 minutes of cycle ergometer exercise at 80% VO2 max. The study was designed to investigate the acute effects of high-intensity exercise on biochemical bone markers. Furthermore, the effect of the oral intake of a 1,000 mg calcium load was checked by giving subjects high-calcium mineral water just prior to and during exercise. The serum concentrations of calcium, phosphate, parathyroid hormone (PTH), bone alkaline phosphatase (BAP), and C-terminal cross-linking telopeptide of type-1 collagen (CTX) were measured before, during, and after exercise. When the exercise was performed without calcium, both serum concentrations and total amount of CTX (a marker of bone resorption) began to increase progressively 30 minutes after the start of exercise and were still elevated by 45–50% two hours post-exercise. Ingestion of the high-calcium mineral water completely suppressed the CTX response. The study appears to demonstrate that the breakdown of bone can be prevented by ingesting calcium prior to exercise.

Based on empirical evidence, experts believe that an ideal pre-exercise meal should:

1. be consumed at least 2–3 hours prior to the start of exercise;
2. contain mainly low or moderate GI carbohydrates;
3. contain minimal fat and protein;
4. be familiar and easily digested;
5. contain a whole food or supplemental source of calcium (300–500 mg); and
6. include ample fluid so that urine is pale prior to the start of exercise.

Examples of good pre-exercise foods include:

- Lentil/bean soup
- Quinoa
- Calcium fortified soy or rice milk
- Barley, rice, or oat grain cereals
- Pasta products (with no/low fat sauce)

- Fruit/vegetable beverages or smoothies
- Sweet potato/yams
- Winter squash (acorn, butternut)
- Applesauce
- Baby food (mixed fruit/vegetable with + / − meat)

If you are not accustomed to eating prior to exercise, especially in the morning, we recommend that you start with a small amount of easily digested food and gradually increase volume. If you are an individual who simply cannot eat in the morning before exercise, we strongly encourage a later exercise time so that you have had the chance to eat prior to exercise. At a minimum, we suggest a calcium and vitamin D supplement with water prior to all exercise sessions regardless of duration or intensity levels. You should make every attempt to precede prolonged or intense sessions with a meal of real food more than two hours prior to the start of exercise. This schedule reduces the likelihood that insulin will contribute to premature fatigue.

The goal of a morning meal is to top off liver glycogen stores, which decrease overnight. During the overnight fast, only liver (not muscle) glycogen levels are reduced. Muscle glycogen levels are largely contingent on your nutritional intake immediately following your last exercise session and are generally well preserved during the overnight fast. This meal does not need to be large, since liver glycogen storage is in the order of 300 kcal.

The average 150-pound male has approximately 1,800–1,900 kcal of carbohydrate storage available in approximately the following distribution:

- Blood glucose (80 kcal)
- Liver glycogen (300 kcal)
- Muscle glycogen (1,500 kcal)

Travel and race anxiety often make digestion more difficult. For these reasons, being familiar with your digestive system's capacity is important, and you should practice your pre-competition meals multiple times during training. Mealtime may need to be slightly modified to match your unique circumstances. Some athletes prefer a pre-exercise meal containing little or no fiber (low residue), while others seem to be particularly sensitive to dairy products or wheat. Many of our athletes have had extremely good results with meals containing sweet potatoes or cooked grains (brown rice, quinoa, oatmeal) mixed with applesauce or bananas.

Many coaches and athletes favor exercising in the fasted state. The rationale for this so-called lipolytic training is to enable athletes to condition themselves to tolerate low blood sugars. Proponents of this philosophy also suggest that training duration may be reduced since blood glucose levels have been decreased by fasting prior to the start of exercise rather than through exercise itself. We acknowledge that in the absence of available glucose, insulin levels are reduced and fatty acid mobilization is enhanced. However, this method of training has the potential to create significant catabolic effects that may result in loss of both lean (muscle) and bone mass. To date, we are unaware of any documented performance benefits that have been attributed to training in the fasted state and therefore do not endorse the concept at this time.

Fueling During Exercise

A well-conditioned athlete who begins exercise with a moderately full tank of muscle and liver glycogen is capable of performing at relatively high intensities for approximately 90–120 minutes. After this time, blood glucose levels decline (hypoglycemia) and performance decays. Beyond two or more hours of high intensity exercise, both carbohydrate and fluid deficits result. Therefore, the aim of fueling during training or competition is to delay fatigue by attempting to maintain blood glucose and fluid levels. Maintenance of glucose and fluid homeostasis supports conservation of bone and lean (muscle) mass as well as minimizes the catabolic effects of cortisol.

Cortisol is a stress hormone that is released from the adrenal glands when blood glucose is low and/or exercise intensity is high. Its purpose is to generate fuel for working muscles. When cortisol is released, it causes the breakdown of protein, carbohydrate, and fat. Elevated cortisol levels create a catabolic effect on body tissues that may offset the anabolic effects of exercise.

Multiple studies have demonstrated that the ingestion of carbohydrate reduces the perception of fatigue and improves performance in prolonged endurance events. Other researchers have reported that carbohydrate ingestion improves high-intensity exercise of short duration (one hour). There is no compelling data to suggest that carbohydrate supplementation improves performance in events lasting 30 minutes or less.

These are our recommendations for carbohydrate and fluid ingestion during exercise:

- Consume 30–80 g (120–320 kcal) of carbohydrate per hour while performing endurance exercise, after the first hour.

- Carbohydrates consumed in liquid, solid, or gel form all have been demonstrated to be equally effective (though individual tolerance varies).

- The rate of carbohydrate absorption decreases in concentrated solutions. Therefore, to optimize carbohydrate and water absorption, carbohydrate solution should be diluted in the 4–8% range for simple sugar solutions such as sports drinks.

- Fructose appears to be oxidized at a lower rate than other simple sugars (glucose, sucrose).

- Multiple carbohydrate sources consumed at the same time may improve the amount of carbohydrate that can be utilized, since each carbohydrate source (glucose, fructose, sucrose, maltodextrin) is transported across the gut wall by separate, noncompetitive pathways.

- The gastric emptying rate may be improved with the use of a glucose polymer (complex carboyhydrate), such as maltodextrin, as compared to simple sugars (glucose, fructose, sucrose).

- Ingestion of 1,000 ml of fluid per hour offsets dehydration during most training or racing conditions and minimizes the likelihood of gastrointestinal distress.

The role of protein in conjunction with supplemental carbohydrate during exercise needs further clarification. To our knowledge, there are no studies that have evaluated bone markers during exercise under conditions of supplemental carbohydrate versus carbohydrate-protein formulas. We do, however, suggest the use of supplemental calcium during prolonged or intense exercise sessions. Although studies are necessary to define dosing recommendations more precisely, 150 mg of calcium per hour of exercise appears to be well tolerated by the athletes who we have worked with. If your preferred source of carbohydrate does not contain calcium, we recommend you consider the addition of supplemental calcium during exercise. Calcium tablets (or chews) can easily be incorporated into a sports drink, mixed into a dehydrated commercial powder/gel, or swallowed along with other (electrolyte) tablets. Whole food sources of calcium that endurance athletes have been known to consume during exercise include chia seeds, figs, raisins, and black strap molasses.

Post-Exercise Nutrition

Following exhausting exercise your body is in a catabolic mode because energy (carbohydrate and fat) and fluid stores have been diminished and somatic tissues (muscle, connective tissue, bone) may be in need of repair. Returning to homeostasis requires food intake. Immediately following exercise (and lasting up to two hours post-exercise), the highest rates of muscle glycogen storage occur, presumably related to increased muscle sensitivity to insulin and glucose as well as the actions of glycogen synthase (Ivy, et al., 1988). Consequently, muscle glycogen storage has been demonstrated to be on the order of 7.7 mmol/kg per hour for the first two hours following exercise, decreasing to approximately 4.3 mmol/kg per hour thereafter (Ivy, et al., 1988). This window is especially important for athletes performing a second exercise session within the next eight hours, since failure to eat during this window may lead to inadequate replenishment for the day's second training session. For athletes engaging in only one training session per day this recovery window may not be as important: Parkin and colleagues (1997) found no difference in glycogen storage at eight and 24 hours post-exercise for athletes consuming carbohydrates immediately following or delaying intake for two hours.

In an excellent review of the literature, Louise Burke and colleagues (2004) have defined what they consider optimal recommendations for carbohydrate intake following exercise. These guidelines are based on the presumption that an endurance athlete's diet should be composed primarily of carbohydrates (60–70%) in order to achieve maximal replenishment of muscle glycogen stores.

- Immediate recovery (0–4 hours): 1.0–1.2 g/kg
- Daily recovery: moderate duration/low intensity training: 5–7 g/kg per day
- Daily recovery: moderate to heavy endurance training: 7–12 g/kg per day
- Daily recovery: extreme exercise program (4–6+ hours per day): 10–12+ g/kg per day

Studies investigating glycogen restoration over 24 hours following exercise show no particular advantage to eating small, frequent meals ("grazing or nibbling") over larger less frequent meals ("gorging"), but many athletes report reduced incidence of GI disturbance with the former.

There is debate about whether low or high GI carbohydrate sources work best during the immediate recovery phase. Some suggest that low GI carbohydrates are superior, while others advocate the converse. Additionally, some studies suggest that a small amount of protein consumed with carbohydrate facilitates glycogen replenishment, but others do not. There is an abundance of references on this subject (Blom, et al., 1987; Ivy, et al., 2002; Jozsi, et al., 1996; Van Loon, et al., 2000; Zachwieja, 2002). Overall, however, the most important determinant of short-term recovery with respect to muscle glycogen appears to be related to the timing and presence of adequate carbohydrate.

Historically, most post-exercise nutritional studies have focused on the rate or degree to which muscle glycogen is restored, but recovery from heavy training or competition is more complex than this. Endurance athletes concerned with musculoskeletal and general health need to consider that post-exercise carbohydrate restoration may be inadequate by itself to realize fully the benefits of their training and minimize bone loss. Among the other processes that proper post-exercise meals may influence are the repair and growth of damaged tissues, the reduction of free radicals, and the recovery of normal immune system and hormonal status. All of these effects will improve subsequent performance.

One of the early studies that demonstrated the importance of timing and protein in post-exercise nutrition was performed on rats by Masashigi Suzuki and colleagues from the University of Wasida in Japan in 1999. These researchers either fed the rats one hour before exercise or delayed feeding for four hours following exercise. The post-exercise meal was composed of high GI carbohydrate and protein in a trial lasting 10 weeks. At the end of the study there was no difference in weight gain between the two groups of animals; however, muscle mass was 6% higher and body fat 25% lower in the group fed one hour post-exercise.

In another study (Stevenson, et al., 2005), a low GI diet following exercise resulted in superior subsequent endurance performance the following day as compared to a diet with high GI content. Nine males participated in two trials. On day 1, subjects ran for 90 minutes at 70% VO2 max. Thereafter, they were supplied with either a high GI or low GI carbohydrate diet which provided 8 g of CHO per kilogram of body mass. On the following day, after an overnight fast, subjects ran to exhaustion at 70% VO2 max. Time to exhaustion was significantly longer in the low GI trial than in the high GI trial. Fat oxidation rates and free fatty acid concentrations were found to be higher during the low GI trial, suggesting that the improvements in endurance were a consequence of increased fat oxidation following the low GI diet.

In a more recent human experiment, Howarth and colleagues (2009) studied response to three different post-exercise nutritional strategies (low carbohydrate, carbohydrate plus protein, high carbohydrate) during the three hours immediately following a two-hour bout of cycle exercise. The low-carbohydrate trial consisted of 1.2 g CHO/kg per hour, the protein plus carbohydrate trial consisted of 1.2 g CHO/kg per hour plus 0.4 g protein/kg per hour, and the high-carbohydrate trial consisted of 1.6 g CHO/kg per hour. The rate of glycogen resynthesis was not different between trials. However, mixed muscle fractional synthetic rate (a measure of muscle synthesis) was increased only in the carbohydrate plus protein trial. This increase in overall net protein synthesis was mainly attributable to a reduced rate of protein catabolism following exercise.

In contrast to the relatively well-studied aspects of recovery nutrition featuring carbohydrate and more recently carbohydrate plus protein, the subject of intramuscular fat restoration following exercise has not yet been well defined. Intramuscular lipid represents a potentially important energy source for human skeletal muscle. Following exhausting exercise this substrate decreases. Its recovery is dependent upon post-exercise nutrition.

Van Loon and colleagues (2003) investigated the effects of endurance exercise and recovery on intramuscular triglyceride (IMTG) content of the vastus lateralis muscle in trained male cyclists. Nine athletes were provided a standard diet for three days, after which they performed a three-hour exercise trial at 55% maximum workload. Before and immediately after exercise, then after 24 and 48 hours of recovery, magnetic resonance spectroscopy (MRS) was performed to measure IMTG content. Muscle biopsies were taken after 48 hours of recovery to determine IMTG content by quantitative fluorescence microscopy. The entire procedure was performed two times; in one trial, a diet containing 39% energy in the form of fat was provided (normal fat, NF) and in the other an athlete's typical carbohydrate-rich diet containing 24% fat (low fat, LF) was provided. During exercise, IMTG content decreased by 21.4 +/- 3.1%. In recovery, IMTG content increased significantly in the normal fat trial only, reaching pre-existing levels within 48 hours. In conclusion, when a normal diet containing approximately 39% fat is ingested during recovery, IMTG content is restored within 48 hours. In contrast, IMTG restoration is impaired substantially when a typical, carbohydrate-rich, athletic diet was used.

Using a randomly assigned crossover design, another research team (Larsen-Meyer, et al., 2002) evaluated the change in intramuscular lipid stores (IMCL, where lipid = triglyceride) from baseline after a two-hour treadmill run (67% VO2 max), along with the recovery of IMCL in response to a post-exercise low fat (10% of energy, LFAT) or moderate fat (35% of energy, MFAT) recovery diet in seven female runners. IMCL was measured in the soleus muscle before, immediately after, and at 22 and 70 hours following the run. Levels of IMCL fell by approximately 25% during the endurance run and were dependent on dietary fat content for post-exercise recovery. Consumption of the MFAT recovery diet allowed IMCL stores to return to baseline by 22 hours and to overshoot (versus baseline) by 70 hours post-exercise. In contrast, consumption of the LFAT recovery diet did not allow IMCL stores to return to baseline even by 70 hours after the run. These results suggest that a certain quantity of dietary fat is required to replenish IMCL after endurance running.

The addition of dietary fat to post-exercise recovery nutrition does not appear to limit carbohydrate or glycogen recovery. In a paper titled "Adding fat calories to meals after exercise does not alter glucose tolerance," Fox and colleagues (2004) reported a novel experiment designed to determine whether adding fat calories to meals after exercise alters glucose tolerance or glycogen synthesis the following day. Seven males cycled 90 minutes at 66% VO2 max followed by a maximum of five high-intensity intervals. During the hours following exercise, the subjects ingested three meals containing either low-fat (5% energy from fat) or high-fat (45% energy from fat) foods. Each diet contained the same amount of protein and carbohydrate. Muscle glycogen and intramuscular triglyceride (IMTG) concentrations were measured in muscle biopsy samples obtained immediately before exercise and the next morning. The day after exercise, muscle glycogen concentration was identical in high-fat and low-fat conditions. At the same time, IMTG concentration was approximately 20% greater during the high-fat compared with the low-fat trial. Despite the addition of approximately 165 g of fat to meals after exercise (approximately 1,500 kcal), glucose tolerance was unchanged. As long as meals ingested in the hours following exercise contain the same carbohydrate content, the addition of approximately 1,500 kcal from fat to these meals did not alter muscle glycogen synthesis or glucose tolerance the next day.

Finally, there has been increased interest in the potential use of cow's milk in sports nutrition. In response to this possibility, Brian Roy from Brock University recently published a review article entitled, "Milk: the new sports drink?" Roy (2008) surveyed the relevant literature, reporting that milk appears to be an effective post-resistance exercise beverage that results in favorable acute alterations in protein metabolism and lean mass. Although research is limited, preliminary reports suggest that low-fat milk has been shown to be as effective, if not more effective, than commercially available sports drinks as a rehydration beverage for endurance athletes. Also exploring this possibility, Karp and colleagues (2006) studied nine endurance-trained cyclists while they performed an interval workout followed by four hours of recovery, and then a subsequent endurance trial to exhaustion at 70% VO2 max, on three separate days. Immediately following the first exercise bout and two hours of recovery, subjects drank equivalent volumes of chocolate milk (70 g carbohydrate, 18 g protein, 5 g fat), fluid replacement drink (water with 30 g carbohydrate), or manufactured carbohydrate replacement drink (70 g carbohydrate, 18 g protein, 1.5 g fat) in single blind randomized design. Time to exhaustion (TTE), average heart rate (HR), rating of perceived exertion (RPE), and total work (WT) for the endurance exercise were compared between trials. TTE and WT were approximately 50% greater for chocolate milk and the manufactured recovery drink as compared to the low carbohydrate fluid replacement. The results of this study suggest that chocolate milk is at least as effective as a commercial recovery product (and may be less expensive!) in short-term recovery between exercise bouts.

Based upon the literature reviewed here, endurance athletes should consider the importance of both protein and fat as well as carbohydrate replacement following exercise. This balanced approach to nutrition departs from the traditional emphasis on carbohydrates alone. As we have discussed in Chapters 5 and 6 on protein and fat, these macronutrients have important implications for bone health as well as the immune system. In addition, the inclusion of moderate amounts of dietary fat appears to enable athletes to counterbalance exercise energy expenditure and protect them from injury. Lastly, a diet that is moderate versus high in carbohydrate seems better to support cardiac health and reduce the likelihood of increasing systemic inflammation, which is the prerequisite for not only bone loss but a host of other degenerative diseases.

Summary

To maximize performance and minimize bone and muscle loss, endurance athletes may consider these important points regarding their nutrition before, during, and after training or competition:

- A pre-exercise meal should be consumed more than 2 hours prior to the start of exercise and contain mostly low to moderate glycemic index carbohydrates (300 kcal).

- The pre-exercise meal should include foods rich in calcium, magnesium, and potassium. Plant-based, whole foods should be an athlete's first choice.

- The pre-exercise meal should be familiar and easily digested. Pre-competition meals should be rehearsed on multiple occasions.

- Urine color should be clear prior to the start of exercise.

- In order to sustain performance for events lasting over 90–120 minutes, supplemental carbohydrate should be consumed at a rate of 30–80 g per hour and fluid intake should be in the range of 1,000 ml/hour.

- We recommend supplemental calcium in the range of 150 mg per hour during prolonged exercise sessions (> 1–2 hours).

- Upon the completion of exercise there is a relatively small window (< 2 hours) for the optimal rate of muscle glycogen re-synthesis to occur. Carbohydrate intake during the hours immediately following exercise is critical for athletes who will participate in a subsequent training session within 8 hours. Additionally, nutritional countermeasures immediately following exercise appear have the greatest opportunity to arrest exercise-induced inflammation and free radical damage as well as optimize body composition.

- There are valuable reasons over and above the restoration of muscle glycogen to include protein and fat in conjunction with carbohydrate during both the immediate and subsequent hours following exercise.

- In the hours immediately following exercise the glycemic index of carbohydrates does not appear to be of significant concern with respect to glycogen restoration. However, beyond two to four hours following exercise, a low glycemic index, plant-based carbohydrate source, combined with adequate protein and fat to counterbalance exercise energy expenditure, appears to maximize health and performance.

- Consider plant-based foods as your primary fuel source, especially those rich in elements known to be protective of bone (including calcium, magnesium, and potassium), in order to limit free radical damage and inflammatory reactions that may lead to skeletal loss.

REFERENCES

Blom PCS, Hostmark AT, Vaage O, Kandel KR, Maehlum S (1987) Effect of different post-exercise sugar diets on the rate of muscle glycogen synthesis. *Medicine and Science in Sports and Exercise* 19:491–496.

Burke LM, Collier GR, Hargreaves M (1993) Muscle glycogen storage after prolonged exercise: effects of the glycemic index of carbohydrate feedings. *Journal of Applied Physiology* 75:1019–1023.

Burke L, Kiens B, Ivy J (2004) Carbohydrates and fat for training and recovery. *Journal of Sports Sciences* 22:15–30.

Chen YJ, Wong SH, Chan CO, Wong CK, Lam CW, Siu PM (2009) Effects of glycemic index meal and CHO-electrolyte drink on cytokinetic response and run performance. *Journal of Science and Medicine in Sport* 12:697–703.

Foster-Powell K, Holt SHA, Brad-Miller JC (2002) International table of glycemic index and glycemic load values. *American Journal of Clinical Nutrition* 76:5–56.

Fox A, Kaufman A, Horowitz J (2004) Adding fat calories to meals after exercise does not alter glucose tolerance. *Journal of Applied Physiology* 97(1):11–16.

Gretebeck RJ, Gretebeck KA, Tittlebach TJ (2002) Glycemic index of popular sports drinks and energy foods. *Journal of the American Dietetics Association* 102(3):415–416.

Guezennec CY, Satabin P, Duforez F, Koziet J, Antoine JM (1993) The role of type and structure of complex carbohydrates on response to physical exercise. *International Journal of Sports Nutrition* 14:224–231.

Guillemant J, Accarie C, Peres G, Guillemant S (2004) Acute effects of an oral calcium load on makers of bone metabolism during endurance cycling exercise in male athletes. *Calcified Tissue International* 74(5): 407–414.

Howarth K, Moreau N, Phillips S, Gibala M (2009) Coingestion of protein with carbohydrate during recovery from endurance exercise stimulates skeletal muscle protein synthesis in humans. *Journal of Applied Physiology* 106(4):1394–1402.

Ivy J, Katz A, Cutler C, Sherman W, Coyle E (1988) Muscle glycogen synthesis after exercise: effect of time of carbohydrate ingestion. *Journal of Applied Physiology* 64:1480–1485.

Ivy J (2001) Dietary strategies to promote glycogen synthesis after exercise. *Canadian Journal of Applied Physiology* 26 (suppl):S236–245.

Ivy J, Goforth H, Damon B, McCauley T, Parsons E, Price T (2002) Early post exercise muscle glycogen recovery is enhanced with a carbohydrate-protein supplement. *Journal of Applied Physiology* 93(4):1337–1344.

Jozsi A, Trappe T, Starling R, Goodpaster B, Trappe S, Fink W, Costill D (1996) The influence of starch structure on glycogen resynthesis and subsequent cycling performance. *International Journal of Sports Medicine* 17:373–378.

Karp J, Johnston J, Tecklenburg S, Mickleborough T, Fly A, Stager J (2006) Chocolate milk as a post-exercise recovery aid. *International Journal of Sports Nutrition and Exercise Metabolism* 16(1):78–91.

Kirwan J, Cyr-Campbell D, Campbell WW, Scheiber J, Evans W (2001) Effects of moderate and high glycemic index meals on metabolism and exercise performance. *Metabolism* 50(7):849–855.

Larsen-Meyer D, Newcomer B, Huner G (2002) Influence of endurance running and recovery diet on intramyocellular lipid content in women: a 1H NMR study. *American Journal of Physiology Endocrinology and Metabolism* 282(1):E95–E106.

Maresh C, Whittlesey M, Armstrong L, Yamamoto L, Judelson D, Fish K, Casa D, Kavouras S, Castracane V (2006) Effect of hydration state on testosterone and cortisol responses to training-intensity exercise in collegiate runners. *International Journal of Sports Medicine* 27(10):765–770.

Parkin J, Carey M, Martin I, Stojanovska L, Febbraio M (1997) Muscle glycogen storage following prolonged exercise: effect of timing of ingestion of high glycemic index food. *Medicine and Science in Sports and Exercise* 29:220–224.

Roy B (2008) Milk: the new sports drink? *Journal of the International Society of Sports Nutrition* 5:15.

Stevenson E, Williams C, McComb G, Oram C (2005) Improved recovery from prolonged exercise following the consumption of low glycemic index carbohydrate meals. *International Journal of Sports Nutrition and Exercise Metabolism* 15(4):333–349.

Suzuki M, Doi T, Lee SJ, Okamura K, Shimuzu S, Okano G, Sato Y (1999) Effect of meal timing after resistance exercise on hind-limb muscle mass and fat accumulation in trained rats. *Journal of Nutritional Science and Vitaminology* 45:401–409.

Thomas D, Brotherhood J, Brand JC (1991) Carbohydrate feeding before exercise: effect of glycemic index. *International Journal of Sports Nutrition* 12:180–186.

Thomas DE, Brotherhood JR, Brand Miller J (1994) Plasma glucose levels after prolonged strenuous exercise correlate inversely with glycemic response to food consumed before exercise. *International Journal of Sports Nutrition* 4:361–373.

Van Loon L, Saris W, Kruijshoop M, Wagenmakers A (2000) Maximizing post-exercise muscle glycogen synthesis: carbohydrate supplementation and the application of amino acid and protein hydrolysate mixtures. *American Journal of Clinical Nutrition* 72:106–111.

Van Loon L, Schrauwen-Hinderling V, Koopman R, Wagenmakers A, Hesselink M, Schaart G, Kooi M, Saris W (2003) *American Journal of Physiology and Endocrinology Metabolism* 285(4):E804–811.

Wright D, Sherman W, Dernbach A (1991) Carbohydrate feedings before, during, or in combination improves cycling endurance performance. *Journal of Applied Physiology* 71(3): 1082–1088.

Zachwieja J (2002) Protein: power or puffery? *Gatorade Sports Science Institute-Sports Science Center. Available:www.gssiweb.com/reflib/refs/338/Protein in Sports Drinks.*

CHAPTER ELEVEN

Quality Training

Years ago, my family doctor told me that if I wished to succeed as a coach and as a runner myself, I would have to consider all factors and not overlook the slightest detail as invariably these were the important ones that made the difference between the successful athlete and the unsuccessful. I have proved this to myself on many occasions and advise all athletes and coaches to also think deeply about their general training plan, daily training sessions, and all factors influencing their lives and those of their athletes.
—Arthur Lydiard in *Runner's Bible*, United States Track and Field Federation, 1970

Training methods promoted for improving endurance performance vary considerably; even "expert" advice is often contradictory. Sir Roger Banister, the first individual to break the four-minute mile barrier, realized his legendary achievement with a program of quarter-mile intervals that required only 30 minutes of training several times per week. At the other end of the spectrum, Arthur Lydiard, the famous New Zealand coach, proposed a steady running regime of over 100 miles per week for his Olympians competing in the half mile. Whether runners should develop endurance prior to speed or use speed to improve endurance, and many similar questions, continue to be debated by athletes and scientists alike.

To improve one's own performance it is crucial to recognize the individual nature of the process. As the running philosopher and physician George Sheehan declared, "Life is the great experiment. Each of us is an experiment of one—observer and subject—making choices, living with them, recording their effects" (*Running & Being*, 1978, p. 138). It is true that no two individuals adapt to a particular program in the same manner. Differences in genetic endowment, personal beliefs, and motivation dictate how an individual athlete responds to training. Additionally, age, training experience, environmental conditions, equipment (or the lack thereof), time, and injury may influence the manner in which one trains. A thorough understanding of exercise physiology and biomechanics is of primary importance for the training of an endurance athlete; but, unlike following a recipe, a single, perfect plan simply does not exist for all athletes at all times.

Despite the fervor with which some advocates promote their own particular approach, there is little scientific support in favor of one training regime over another. This is especially true for the "mature" or well-trained athlete, since much of the published exercise physiology literature is gleaned from investigations of college-aged males—often active, but largely untrained. A good starting point for anyone seeking to understand these complications in formulating an effective, personalized training protocol is the excellent review by Kubukeli and colleagues on the scientific studies that have examined endurance training protocols and the tapering process ("Training techniques to improve endurance exercise performances," 2002). Additional insight into the limits of human performance are offered in the articles "Mind and muscle: The cognitive-affective neuroscience of exercise" by Stein and colleagues (2007) and "The limits of endurance exercise" by Noakes (2006).

Although some would argue that genetics is responsible for optimal performance, there are many stories of athletes with substandard natural endowments outperforming more gifted competitors. Likewise, simply "working harder" is not the answer, as history is filled with stories of athletes who have achieved greatness on scant training and those that have been destroyed by doing too much.

In *The Lore of Running*, Tim Noakes, MD, recommends that you achieve as much as possible on a minimum of training (his Law 6). In brief, there is a limit to the amount of training from which the body can benefit. Many athletes are under the impression that the more they train the greater their degree of improvement will be. But the law of diminishing returns is very operational in the world of endurance training.

Bruce Fordyce, world record holder and one of history's most decorated ultramarathon runners, attributed much of his success to the fact that he rarely did too much and emphasized rest and recovery. In 1981 he wrote, "I do believe in hard training, but there is only so much hard training that the body can take." Fordyce recognized early in his career that running success was not contingent on training volume. Consequently, he spent a substantial amount of his training year dedicated to shorter distance track racing (1,500–10,000 meter distances), which he believed helped him achieve a faster "cruising speed" for ultramarathons.

A common mantra is that 80% of endurance performance is determined by only 20% of your training. If this rule of thumb is correct, a great percentage of training time may be responsible for a small percentage of return—or, worse yet, may contribute to an actual decline in performance. For this reason, any individual who is interested in maximizing performance while minimizing bone loss must grasp the paramount importance of understanding how to prioritize training.

We believe that an effective training program must be designed with the individual in mind. It should emphasize overcoming personal limitations as well as developing technical skill and perception. As Rene Descartes stated, "It is not enough to have a good mind. The main thing is to use it well."

The identification of personal limitations is challenging for the self-coached athlete, who may be better served through an assessment by a qualified mentor or trainer. For example, in the clinic we often identify endurance athletes with strength and balance deficits, both of which can significantly limit endurance performance and/or increase the likelihood of injury. Strength and balance can be tested in a variety of ways, but practical strength tests include the single-leg squat and single-arm push-up (Tsatsouline, 2004), while static balance can be assessed by a series of single-leg standing tests.

Self-testing can be a good starting point. To test your basic balance, try the following three test(s). Testing should be performed on a level surface with no shoes.

1. Stand on one foot with the opposite lower extremity raised and positioned next to the weight-bearing knee. Cross your arms over your chest and focus your eyes straight ahead. Your pelvis should remain level. Your goal is to maintain balance for 10 seconds. The test outcome is considered positive if you do not lose your neutral hip alignment, need to touch the floor with your non-weight bearing leg, or move your arms from their starting position. Both sides should be tested, since subtle differences between sides may be relevant. If you can pass test number one easily, advance to the next level.

2. Test position is the same, but the goal is to maintain balance while slowly rotating your head and neck from left to right (maximal rotation should be achieved as if you are attempting to look behind your shoulder). Your goal is to maintain standing balance for the duration of time required to perform four side-to-side repetitions

of the head rotation. If this result is achieved, advance to the next level.

3. The final test in this progression of balance is to maintain the single-leg balance while closing your eyes. The goal is to maintain balance for more than 10 seconds. Studies have demonstrated that the failure to successfully perform this test for at least 10 seconds accurately predicts injury in a population of high school and collegiate athletes (Trojian and McKeag, 2006; Levinger, et al., 2007).

It can be very enlightening for endurance athletes to appreciate just how much better their performance can be if they achieve basic balance and stability. Visualize the balance and ease with which world-class endurance athletes move. Human movement can be reduced to basic postures, or what Dr. Nicholas Romanov calls "poses." If you lack the strength and balance to maintain stability in the basic static postures and the skill to transition and repeat, dynamic performance will be surely compromised. Visualize how necessary this single-leg balance position is for efficient running, cycling, or even rowing.

This simple concept "balance" also may have larger implications. Marian Wolfe Dixon, in her book *Bodylessons: Exploring the Wisdom of Your Body,* has made thoughtful observations regarding physical and emotional balance:

> Right now, take a moment to stand up and balance on one leg. If it is easy for you to balance, do so with your eyes closed. Make a mental note of how easy or difficult it is for you to do. The next time you are "upset," either with anger, sadness, or another emotion, see if you can disengage yourself enough to explore the effect of the upset emotions on your body. You can do this by re-administering the above-mentioned balance test. If you continue to think about how upset you are it will be relatively difficult to balance. On the other hand, if you concentrate on balancing, you may find yourself feeling less upset. Physical and emotional balance go hand in hand. Emphasis on one exerts an influence on the other. (74)

In addition to becoming a student of your chosen endurance pursuit and consulting knowledgeable professionals or peers regarding the pillars of physical training, as an athlete you should strive to cultivate not only technical skill but also the relationship between mind and body. As Tim Noakes (2006:417) has written, "For it is the mind that determines who chooses to start and who best stays the distance."

Martial arts master Bruce Kumar Frantzis provided the following insight in Jess O'Brien's excellent internal martial arts book, *Nei Jia Quan* (2007:172):

At each stage every external movement has inner forms and outer forms. Your outer, external form is where your torso, head, arms, and legs are moving through space. Your inner form is what you are doing inside your body with your mind and with your energy. Your awareness of how little body parts move is also part of the inner form. Most people in the West are not terribly aware of inner forms. And if you're going to go from the stage of form to no form, everything in this form has to become awake before you can drop it. You have to know how to ride a bike before you can forget about it and just ride. There's no free lunch, although lots of people...fantasize that there is. The nature of a specific situation determines how the various training methods are done with all the minor details. The minor details are all the important details. The most talented have the natural ability to see something and make all the parts just come together. Others get it better by clearly being taught in very specific, articulated detail.

In our opinion there is more to gain by learning, perceiving, and refining exercise technique than through perhaps any other single element of endurance training. The value of dedicating yourself to becoming a student of technique has the potential to provide benefits in several ways, including:

- enabling you to focus your mental and physical energies in purposeful rather than wasteful directions;
- providing a vehicle for qualitative versus quantitative assessment of training and racing; and
- facilitating the integration of mental and physical realms that define optimal experience and performance.

Many individuals do not recognize the skill that is required to succeed in endurance athletics or that technique can be learned. There is a prevailing attitude among many athletes that to become a "better" runner, cyclist, or swimmer, all that is necessary is to train more. Sadly, this is not the case; history is filled with stories of athletes who have increased training volumes and performed at or below their previous levels. We believe that improved exercise technique is not merely the result of high-volume training, but rather the result of focused efforts.

For any endurance activity there are certain fundamental biomechanical principles that govern movement. Unfortunately, most endurance athletes do not understand how to apply and integrate their muscular efforts in a manner that is consistent with these principles. The integration of voluntary muscular actions with biomechanics is complicated; for most athletes, just describing how their bodies interact with the natural environment or with their equipment is a challenge. To illustrate the point, complete these two simple exercises and then ask your peers or coach to do the same:

1. Describe the mechanics of an elite distance runner.

2. To increase running speed, I . . .

What challenges are posed here? Are your responses similar to or different from those of your teammates or coach? The fact that many athletes find this exercise difficult illustrates the lack of information with which most endurance athletes are operating. Without a solid understanding of movement principles, athletes have a difficult time learning and mastering their craft and may be emotionally disconnected from their physical selves. The results are wasted physical and emotional energy and an insufficient ability to develop focus and concentration.

Consider the difference between a bar room brawler and a highly skilled martial artist or boxer. In a fight, the bar room brawler will work hard, expend enormous amounts of energy, and perhaps land an occasional punch. The trained fighter is a calm, emotional center, capable of yielding and attacking with a perfect blend of relaxation and tension; energy expenditure is consistent with demands and movements appear automatic and effortless.

Most of us can appreciate the technical competence required for "highly skilled" sports such as gymnastics, martial arts, or fencing. But technical competence is unappreciated in endurance sports. Many endurance athletes, especially Americans, seem to concern themselves with the physiological aspects of performance and do not address the technical, psychomotor, or perceptual components of training. In his book *Running Fast and Injury Free* (edited by Dr. John S. Gilbody, available free online), Gordon Pirie states, "Before you have taught yourself to train properly, you must become conscious of the necessity of running properly and take steps towards developing correct technique. The best training in the world will be worthless if proper technique is not employed. This vital factor in a runner's development is all but ignored by most coaches."

Endurance athletes who fully appreciate the basis for the skill of human movement will have enhanced perception and can recognize dysfunctional versus functional actions. Until an athlete has the opportunity to experience and identify these sensations, there is no basis for comparison; refinement of technique, if there is any, is accidental or sporadic.

Swimming, for example, is a sport that most people recognize as requiring at least a basic level of technical competence. However, the current standard for most developmental swimming programs is that participants should swim great distances with the assumption that "proper" stroke mechanics will simply evolve as the laps accumulate. In many programs, young children swim distances of 5,000–7,000 meters per day in practice (using primarily aerobic metabolic pathways) in preparation for race events that are anaerobic in nature and only 50–100 meters in length. Generally, little or no attention is devoted to the development of sound technique. This approach is in sharp contrast to the level of technical instruction provided to budding figure skaters, gymnasts, or tennis players.

A recent article in the *New York Times Magazine* detailing the famed Dutch Soccer Club Ajax underscores the importance of this point. Ruben Jongkind, a consultant who works mainly with Dutch track athletes, was observed altering the posture and running gait of a 15-year-old soccer player. Jongkind reportedly said, "While the boy was actually quite fast, he did not have enough range of motion in his vertical plane and was running like a duck, shuffling." Jongkind continued, "That takes more energy, which is why we have to change his motor patterns, so he can be as fast at the end of a game as the beginning." The coach had been working with this particular player for several weeks and said that he had progressed to be "consciously able but not subconsciously able" to run with the desired form, meaning that in the heat of competition, he reverted to his old form.

Consider this question: If one of the most respected developmental soccer programs in the world considers it important enough to consult with running specialists to ensure that their soccer players are developing proper running form, don't you think it stands to reason that our running (or swimming, cycling, rowing) programs should invest at least as much attention to the subject?

Terry Laughlin, swimming coach and founder of Total Immersion Swimming has this to say:

> After 38 years of purposeful swimming and 32 years of coaching and teaching, I think I'm fortunate to have achieved a rare distinction: I think I have become one of the best swimmers on earth. While that claim probably sounds staggeringly presumptuous, my definition of "best"—unlike one that applies to, say, Michael Phelps—doesn't hinge on how fast I swim. Instead I mean that, among the billions in the human race, there are perhaps only a hundred or so swimmers on earth who use their available energy and power as efficiently as I do, who enjoy every stroke as fully and who practice effectively enough to keep improving continuously.

It's that last definition of "best" that excites me the most. There's a Japanese term "Kaizen" which means continuous improvement; specifically it infers "incremental improvement through cleverness, patience and diligence." At age 53, I feel I'm the embodiment of Kaizen swimming. I'm still making regular advances in my control, efficiency, and ease. I also swim 1500 meters faster than I did as an 18-year old college freshman in 1969.

The only time my swimming stagnated was my final two years of college—when I believed that working hard was the way to success. From the time I began swimming as a high school sophomore through my college years I prided myself on working harder than anyone else in the pool and—for a few years—I improved steadily. I also swam an average of 40,000 yards per week (compared to 15,000 now) and was a lean and hungry teenager. But in my final two years of college, I continued working hard and actually regressed. In fact it was that frustration as an athlete that led me into coaching.

Over the 32 years since college I've stopped concentrating on how hard and shifted to a focus on achieving flow while in the pool and improved each year without pause. If you'd like to achieve a similar Nirvana, here are the rules for Kaizen Swimming:

- Working hard doesn't help
- Swimming your best doesn't hurt
- Be the quiet center
- Pay attention to yourself
- Never push off without a plan

(http://www.beginnertriathlete.com/TerryLaughlin/kaizen_swimming.htm; used with the author's permission)

For more of Terry Laughlin's perspective and philosophy, visit www.totalimmersion.net.

The development of sport-specific techniques are beyond the scope of this book, but there are some general guidelines for cultivating excellence that are nearly universal. What do Kenyan distance runners, Brazilian soccer players, and Russian tennis players have in common with some of histories greatest writers, artists, and chess players? For an in-depth look at the topic of cultivating excellence, we highly recommend *The Talent Code,* by Daniel Coyle. Coyle is also the author of *Lance Armstrong's War.*

It turns out that one of the most important methods in the cultivation of excellence is to define a reference standard, a "benchmark" or intended target from which you can compare your present status.

You might make a video analysis or careful observation of the world's elite endurance athletes. Once you have identified such a standard of reference, you need to fully understand all of its component parts and how they relate to each other as part of a larger whole.

As the whole takes shape, challenging yourself by working at different speeds becomes important. Depending upon the nature of the sport or the intended purpose of the training session, the alteration in speed may be achieved by increases in cadence or force or combinations of both. Lower-intensity training provides athletes with a non-threatening physiological environment from which they can more closely attend to errors—and these errors are precisely what you are constantly looking to identify. The perception of these "deviations from the standard" and, most important, your timely attempt to resolve them, is precisely the type of training on which your learning centers thrive. Increases in training speed (or durations) are then governed by keen observation of technical errors and their resolution.

Once technical performance starts to decay, perhaps as a result of attempts to go faster, use greater force, or go longer distances, it is time to consider how best to resolve the situation. With thoughtful analysis, you can gain clarity about how best to advance your training and focus your efforts on your unique limitations. It is very interesting to explore this question as frequently performance tends to be limited by mental or emotional rather than physical factors.

We strongly recommend the resource *Programmed to Run* by Thomas Miller. Dr. Miller is a self-described "blue-collar coach" and is a recognized expert in performance enhancement for endurance sports, both in technique and motivation. He is a former Marine, has participated in more than 100 marathons, and has earned a doctorate in exercise and sport science with an emphasis on performance psychology. (We would be remiss if we failed to thank him for revealing his practice of playing with G.I. Joe dolls in the bathtub! Thanks, Tom.) In his book, Dr. Miller provides sound explanations of field-tested strategies runners can use to improve both emotional and biomechanical components of running. An additional reference that provides what we consider the gold standard of "chunk" analysis for swimming, cycling, and running, is Dr. Nicholas Romanov's book, *Pose Method of Triathlon Techniques.*

To achieve the highest quality of life in all of its various pursuits, including endurance training and racing, you must cultivate a purposeful and thoughtful investment in the process rather than just the outcome. As Friedrich von Schiller stated, "Only those who have the patience to do difficult things perfectly will acquire the skill to do difficult things easily."

We believe that meticulous attention to the development of sound technique will provide the basis for long-term development and improvements in both speed and fatigue resistance. In addition to the development of mind-body focus and technical competence, we often suggest to the self-coached athlete (or the coach in charge of a number of athletes with different capability levels) monitoring training status with a model of distance (power or speed also work well) versus time. Distance, power, or speed should be placed on the vertical axis and time on the horizontal axis. A "golden standard" must then be constructed from which you can compare your personal results.

The reference curve can be based on the records or results from a certain class of athletes (club, state, national, Olympic) or the personal records of an athlete you wish to emulate. Triathletes may also consider plotting their individual racing splits (swim, bike, run) as well as their transition times and compare them to a standard.

For example, a middle distance high school swimmer (400 meter) looking to advance to next year's state championships may be plotting a curve based on the results from the previous years' state champions. The winning times from the state meet at distances from 50 meters to 1,500 meters should be plotted and compared to the swimmer's current times. If the percentage of difference between the two curves is greatest in the shorter distances (50 and 100 meters), increasing speed is the priority. Conversely, if the percentage of difference is greatest in the longer distance events (800 and 1,500 meters), training that emphasizes endurance or fatigue resistance is most likely to improve the overall performance to a higher degree.

The current Olympic records for running distances of 200 meters to the marathon are listed in Table 11.1. If you are a distance runner, can you identify your greatest personal strengths and weaknesses? Would you be better served by focusing on developing speed or improving endurance?

Another benefit of monitoring your performance standards throughout the continuum is that it enables you to compare your level of development (or decline) over your career. We consistently meet aging endurance athletes who complain of progressively poorer race results, particularly in the marathon. Often their frustration leads them to increase overall running mileage, which appears to induce further declines in performance and even injury. A speed versus time graph (particularly over several years) almost universally reveals that the most significant decay in performance is at the shorter distances (200–1,500 meters). Armed with this knowledge, training can focus at these distances, which generally improves marathon race performances to a much greater degree than does running additional mileage.

Table 11.1 Olympic records, and yours, for running events

Olympic records	Personal records	Percentage of difference
(200) 19.30		
(400) 43.49		
(800) 1.42.58		
(1,500) 3.32.07		
(5K) 12.57.82		
(10K) 27.01.17		
(42K) 2.06.32		

Summary

The development of a human endurance athlete may be more of an art than a science. Examination of the training programs of both elite and recreational athletes provides evidence that there is no one-size-fits-all approach.

Historically, most endurance athletes have concerned themselves with training volume and intensity and tend continually to train their relative strengths. The motivation to seek and to identify personal limitations, as well as the willingness to resolve them, is emotionally challenging for some and difficult physically for others. Performance limitations may be related to genetic, anthropometric, physiologic, psychological, or technical factors. The aspect of development that is most often overlooked by endurance athletes is what Dr. Thomas Miller defines as the "psychomechanical."

Perhaps the single most important requirement for improving technique is to identify a standard or benchmark from which technical errors can be identified. Consider the difficulty a music student would have in learning a classic piece if he or she never were able to hear it performed at the highest level. Accordingly, observation of elite endurance athletes training or competing (in person or on video) is a valuable instructional instrument. Many athletes are capable of improving their technique simply by emulating the elites. The effectiveness of imitation is one reasons certain geographic locations tend to produce an unusually high percentage of "gifted performers."

With technical excellence as a cornerstone of performance, coaches or movement professionals can help athletes identify precise factors that interfere with the acquisition of superior technique. Common examples of deficits that limit technique and thus performance are shoulder flexibility in swimmers, lower extremity stability and balance in cyclists, and ankle flexibility and elasticity in runners. These deficits generally can be improved with targeted supplemental exercise strategies.

Athletes must cultivate their sense of perception in order to develop psychomotor skills. In other words, it is essential for them to be able to sense when they are performing proper technique and when they are not. The detection of errors or deviations from the standard should be embraced, as it is the recognition of these errors that provides the best stimulus for learning or development. For example, we work with many runners who land on their heels with straight knees. We have them perform the simple exercise of removing their shoes and lightly "bouncing" on the balls of their feet with their knees bent and relaxed. They immediately appreciate the reduction in impact. It is this direct comparison that is so valuable. Assisting an athlete in recognizing, through their own perceptions, how their current technique deviates from that of the intended or gold standard is an important way to enhance their learning.

The transfer of these new perceptions and movement skills provides a means to enrich the training experience. Not only the heightened perceptions and skills, but also one's awareness of these elements, make it possible to achieve new levels of concentration that further enhance alignment of mind and body. With mind and body uniting in a focused manner, distractions such as anxiety and fatigue, which commonly impede performance, become less limiting.

Identification of performance limitations may be further assessed by the construction and analysis of a speed-versus-time graph. The results of this curve can help coaches and athletes achieve a successful balance between speed and endurance training as well as monitor an athlete's long-term development.

REFERENCES

Coyle D (2009) *The Talent Code.* New York: Bantam Dell division. Random House, Inc.

Descartes R (1637) *Le Discours de la Methode* (Discourse on Method and Meditations) translated by LJ Lafleur. New York: The Liberal Arts Press.

Dixon MW (2005) *Bodylessons Exploring the Wisdom of Your Body by Marian Wolfe Dixon.* Edited by Shari Mueller. Forres, Scotland: Findhorn Press.

Fordyce B (1981) *Bruce Fordyce's Comrades Training: The Distance Runners Log.* Pietermaritzburg: Collegian Harriers.

Kubukeli Z, Noakes T, Dennis S (2002) Training techniques to improve endurance exercise performances. *Sports Medicine* 32(8):489–509.

Levinger P, Gilleard W, Coleman C (2007) Femoral medial deviation angle during a one-legged squat test in individuals with patellofemoral pain syndrome. *Physical Therapy in Sport* 8(4):163–168.

Lydiard A (1970) *Runner's Bible.* United States Track and Field Federation.

Miller T (2002) *Programmed to Run.* Champaign, IL: Human Kinetics.

Noakes TD (2003) *The Lore of Running.* 4th ed. Champaign, IL: Human Kinetics.

Noakes T (2006) The limits of endurance exercise. Basic Res Cardiol. 101(5):408–417.

O'Brien J (2007) *Nei Jia Quan Internal Martial Arts.* 2nd edition. Berkley, CA: Blue Snake Books.

Pirie G (2009) *Running Fast and Injury Free.* Ed. Gilbody JS. www.booktraining.net/2009/04/1oo1-books-you-must-have.html.

Romanov N (2008) *Pose Method of Triathlon Techniques.* Coral Gables, FL: Pose Tech Press.

Sokolove M (2010) How a soccer star is made. The *New York Times Magazine.* www.nytimes.com/2010/06/06.

Stein D, Collins M, Daniels W, Noakes T, Zigmond M (2007) Mind and muscle: the cognitive-affective neuroscience of exercise. *CNS Spectrum* 12(1):19–22.

Trojian T, McKeag D (2006) Single leg balance test to identify risk of ankle sprains. *British Journal of Sports Medicine* 40(7):610–613.

Tsatsouline P (2004) *The Naked Warrior* (DVD). St. Paul, MN: Dragon Door Publications.

CHAPTER TWELVE

Measurement of Bone

Why are so many endurance athletes unaware of bone loss until the point of fracture? In short, they don't know until it is too late. Bone loss is an asymptomatic process that may begin months or years before an actual fracture. For this reason, endurance athletes should consider diagnostic testing to monitor their skeletal health. Bone density is a strong predictor of future fracture risk, since density accounts for the majority of bone strength.

Several different tests are available that directly quantify bone mineral density. The gold standard among them is the *dual energy X-ray absorptiometry* (DEXA) scan. Other tests, which are simpler and less expensive, provide data that correlate strongly with DEXA results. Finally, there are laboratory tests available that provide information regarding the remodeling status of the skeleton.

Commercially available DEXA scanners can measure bone mineralization in the spine, femur, forearm, heel, and whole body. The most common measurement sites are the lumbar spine and femur. Measurements from the spine provide a good representation of whole body bone mass; the femur is a common fracture site in senile osteoporosis. In the lumbar spine, measurements usually are taken from each of four lumbar vertebrae (L1–L4), while femoral measurements include the femoral neck, greater trochanter, Ward's triangle, and parts of the femoral shaft.

A DEXA scanner casts two X-ray beams with differing energy levels through bone. Bone mineral density is estimated by the amount of radiation that is absorbed by bone. This result is divided by the area of bone being scanned. Because a DEXA scan result is a calculation of bone mineral density that uses area rather than an actual measurement of volume, it is not entirely accurate. To distinguish

DEXA measures of bone mineral density from a true measurement of volumetric bone mineral density, researchers sometimes refer to the former as "area BMD." DEXA test results also have been reported to overestimate the bone mineral density of taller individuals and underestimate the density of children's bones. Despite these limitations, DEXA test results are still considered to be relatively precise.

Other imaging tests, such as computed quantitative computer tomography (QCT), are capable of measuring bone volume directly and therefore are not susceptible to the confounding effect of bone size. QCT can be used to measure both axial (spinal) and peripheral bones and provides information on both bone density and geometry. These scanners are used mainly in research settings but may be helpful in certain clinical situations in order to differentiate trabecular from cortical bone loss.

Ultrasound densitometry is another commonly utilized test for the measurement of bone density. The ultrasound machine is portable, inexpensive, and involves no radiation. This test may be administered routinely in a physician's office or community health setting. Its main drawback is that it cannot be used to assess bone mass of the spine or femur. The site most commonly measured is the heel because these measurements correlate with spine and femur density as well as with fracture risk. However, for athletes at risk, ultrasound screening should not be considered as a DEXA substitute. This is especially true for runners, who land on their heels.

A bone density test reports the amount of bone mineral that is present within a certain area of bone. Bone mineral density is reported as grams per square centimeter, or g/cm^2. The T-score, a measure of the standard deviation from the average, compares your bone density with that of the average healthy adult. If you have a positive T-score, your bone density is greater than average. If your T-score is greater than -1, your bone mass is within 1 standard deviation of the healthy young adult average, which is considered adequate. T-scores between -1 and -2.5 indicate that your bone mass is lower than normal, and you will be diagnosed with osteopenia. A T-score less than -2.5 means that your bone mass is more than 2.5 standard deviations below that of the average young adult and you are considered to have osteoporosis. Statistically speaking, a T-score of less than -2.5 means your bone density is lower than 99 percent of healthy young adults, so your fracture risk is approximately three times higher than average.

As we age, some bone mineral generally is lost, so there is a tendency for an individual's T-score to decline over the lifetime. A Z-score is a means to describe your bone mass relative to individuals of similar age. The same standard deviations are used, but with a

Z-score the standard of reference comprises individuals of the same age. If your Z-score is decreasing over time, your bone mass is deteriorating more rapidly than would expected as a result of age.

The physician or health care provider who ordered the tests should explain your individual test results in detail. However, if you wish to gain some background in order to understand the results more fully yourself, numerous textbooks of basic statistics are available. A basic example is *Statistics in Kinesiology* (Vincent, 2005); more advanced sources also are available, including online (such as www.statsoft.com). You should be aware that, aside from the statistical measures themselves, there are numerous potential complications in the interpretation of DEXA scores. Carey and colleagues (2007) found that some younger adults (premenopausal women and men under 50 years of age) have larger than expected differences between their DEXA T-scores and Z-scores. In 11% of cases the difference was one standard deviation or more. These differences are due in part to the fact that there is no single standard Z-score definition among diagnostic equipment manufacturers. Factors of this sort should be considered whenever there are differences in successive test results, particularly if they are done by different medical facilities.

Although DEXA scanning is currently the best method available to evaluate bone mineral density and to monitor chronic or long-term changes in the skeleton, because it captures a "snapshot" representation of bone mass the test does not provide any information regarding the extent or direction of skeletal remodeling.

Net bone loss resulting in osteoporosis is characterized both by an imbalance of bone cell activity in which resorption exceeds formation and by increased activation of the entire remodeling process. The rate of formation or degradation of bone can be assessed by measuring enzymatic activity of the bone forming or resorbing cells, as well as by measuring bone matrix components that are released into circulation during remodeling events. These products are known collectively as biochemical markers. Markers can be classified as either resorptive or formative. Because remodeling of bone is a linked or "coupled" event in which resorption proceeds formation, either marker type will reflect to a certain degree the overall remodeling rate. However, the relative degrees to which these two types of bone cells are operating depend upon a variety of factors. If the overall rate of resorption exceeds formation, net bone loss ensues. If formation exceeds resorption, bone mass and strength are gained (see Table 12.1).

For example, as we have discussed in Chapter 4 on metabolism and energy balance, the early stages of an energy deficit are characterized by a reduction in bone formation with stable levels of resorption.

Table 12.1 Biochemical markers of bone turnover

Marker	Type	Specimen
Bone alkaline phosphatase	Formation	Serum (blood)
Osteocalcin	Formation	Serum
Terminal propeptides of type-I procollagen	Formation	Serum
Deoxypridinoline	Resorption	Urine
Hydroxyproline	Resorption	Urine
Telopeptides of type-I collagen	Resorption	Serum/Urine

However, if the energy deficit is increased, resorption rates become elevated, producing an accelerated rate of bone loss. Because bone remodeling is dynamic and the ratio of resorption to formation is variable, analysis of biochemical markers may provide a more useful means to determine the current status of an athlete's skeletal metabolism.

Analyzing bone-remodeling rates can be challenging because they have a circadian rhythm (bone resorption rates generally are elevated at night and during the early morning hours) and are altered by a variety of factors (energy status, nutritional state, hormonal levels, exercise). Biochemical marker tests are most likely to be diagnostically informative for an individual when they are collected in a serial manner by a laboratory specializing in their analysis.

Hetland and colleagues (1993) evaluated 120 males (19–56 years old) who were engaged in variable levels of running (0–160 km/week). The investigators found that bone mineral content at all sites correlated negatively with the distance run weekly. Additionally, the biochemical markers of bone turnover were 20–30% higher in the elite runners, suggesting accelerated bone loss.

The current consensus is that DEXA scanning need not be performed any more frequently than once every two years, even if an athlete is considered to be at high risk for bone loss. This frequency was established because changes in the actual density of bone often cannot be appreciated within shorter time frames. For athletes who have been diagnosed with osteopenia or osteoporosis, however, biochemical markers can be analyzed more frequently. For example, there may be some value in repeating these tests after three months of improved nutritional status and/or hormonal supplementation. Alternatively, it may be prudent to perform baseline tests during an athlete's off-season and then again during a building or high-volume phase in order to ensure that bone turnover is controlled or stable.

Summary

Dual energy absorptiometry (DEXA) provides the current gold standard of estimating bone density. A full DEXA test generally provides information regarding the status of the lumbar spine, hip, and forearm. Test results are reported as T- and Z-scores. T-scores compare your individual results to that of a normal young adult population and Z-scores are based on a comparison to normal, age-matched peers. DEXA tests generally are not repeated any more frequently than once every two years.

The dynamic nature of bone remodeling may be captured through the use of biochemical markers of bone metabolism. Our preferred analyses include bone-specific alkaline phosphatase (BAP), type I collagen propeptide (PICP), and both serum (blood) and urine type I collagen N-telopeptides (NTX). BAP and PICP indicate bone formation whereas NTX is an index of resorption.

Athletes who are concerned about the status of their skeleton may consider discussing with their primary care physician the value of performing these tests to establish a baseline and/or in a serial manner. If bone-remodeling rates appear elevated or if low levels of formation are detected, repeated testing may be useful following treatment interventions. Serial analysis of biochemical markers may assist with the fine-tuning of treatment strategies. Additionally, high-risk athletes may consider having these tests performed throughout the training year as a means to confirm that bone remodeling is remaining stable.

REFERENCES

Beck-Jensen J, Kollerup G, Sorensen H, Pors Nielsen S, Sorensen O (1997) A single measurement of biochemical markers of bone turnover has limited utility in the individual person. *Scandinavian Journal of Clinical Laboratory Investigation* 57(4):351–359.

Bonnick SL, Shulman S (2006) Monitoring osteoporosis therapy: bone mineral density, bone turnover markers, or both? *American Journal of Medicine* 119(4), Supplement 1:S25–S31.

Boppart M, Kimmel D, Yee J, Cullen D (1998) Time course of osteoblast appearance after in vivo mechanical loading. *Bone* 23(5):409–415.

Brahm H, Strom H, Piehl-Aulin K, Mallmin H, Ljunghall S (1997) Bone metabolism in endurance trained athletes: a comparison to population-based controls based on DXA, SXA, quantitative ultrasound, and biochemical markers. *Calcified Tissue International* 61(6):448–454.

Carey JJ, Delaney MF, Love TE, Richmond BJ, Cromer BA, Miller PD, Manilla-Mcintosh M, Lewis SA, Thomas CL, Licata AA (2007) DXA-generated z-scores and t-scores may differ substantially and significantly in young adults. *Journal of Clinical Densitometry* 10(4):351–358.

Creighton D, Morgan A, Boardley D, Brolinson G (2001) Weight-bearing exercise and markers of bone turnover in female athletes. *Journal of Applied Physiology* 90:565–570.

Cunningham J, Segre G, Slatopolsky E, Avioli L (1985) Effects of heavy exercise on mineral metabolism and calcium regulating hormones in humans. *Calcified Tissue International* 37:598–601.

Delmas P, Eastell R, Garnero P, Seibel M, Stepan J (2000) The use of biochemical markers of bone turnover in osteoporosis. *Osteoporosis International* Suppl. 6:S2–17.

Greenspan S, Dresner-Pollak R, Parker R, London D, Ferguson L (1997) Diurnal variation of bone mineral turnover in elderly men and women. *Calcified Tissue International* 60:419–423.

Hetland M, Haarbo J, Christiansen C (1993) Low bone mass and high bone turnover in male long distance runners. *Clinical Endocrinology and Metabolism* 77:770–775.

Notomi T, Okazki Y, Okimoto N, Saitoh S, Nakamura T, Suzuki M (2000) A comparison of resistance and aerobic training for mass, strength and turnover of bone in growing rats. *European Journal of Applied Physiology* 83:469–474.

Vincent W (2005) *Statistics in Kinesiology*, 3rd edition. Champaign, IL: Human Kinetics.

Welsh L, Rutherford O, James I, Crowley C, Comer M, Wolman R (1997) The acute effects of exercise on bone turnover. *International Journal of Sports Medicine* 18:247–251.

CHAPTER THIRTEEN

Stress Fractures

Stress fractures of the skeleton are common injuries that result when microscopic damage to bone exceeds the rate at which it can be remodeled. Stress fractures can have various causes. These influences are not independent of each other, and indeed are more likely to be multiplicative rather than additive; one factor can predispose an athlete to still others.

Risk factors often are categorized as intrinsic or extrinsic. Intrinsic factors are inherent characteristics of the athlete, while extrinsic factors are related to the athlete's environmental circumstances. Intrinsic considerations commonly are due to the expression of genes during development; for example, the relative lengths of the metatarsals or a leg true length inequality. Other examples are alterations in lower extremity alignment as a result of a former traumatic injury. Extrinsic influences include environmental circumstances such as running surface, footwear, or training programs.

Basically, a stress fracture is a bone injury that results from the inability of a bone to withstand repetitive sub-threshold loading. Loads or stresses that act on bones during exercise are related to muscle contractions and ground reaction forces. These stresses result in small bone deformations known as strains. The resultant changes in bone shape are tiny and therefore measured in terms of *microstrain*. Typical values for the loading of bones are in the 100–1,500 microstrain range, whereas strains that are necessary to cause failure in a single load are on the order of 10,000 microstrain. Strains well below the single-load threshold are capable of creating bone damage when introduced in a repetitive or cyclic manner. Such damage is of little significance if repair and remodeling mechanisms are adequate. However, if bone damage exceeds the rate at which it can be repaired and replaced, a bone injury may develop.

Clinically, bone injuries exist on a continuum. A repetitive stress injury generally presents subtly as a state of minimal disruption in the micro-architecture of bone. If training continues and the injury is allowed to progress, the magnitude of the injury increases and it may become in an overt or complete fracture. The very early or embryonic stage of a bone injury is known clinically as a "stress reaction" rather than a stress fracture. At this stage, generally there is no visible fracture line on diagnostic scans. When a fracture line can be identified on a radiograph or other diagnostic scan (MRI), fracture is the preferred diagnostic term.

Stress reaction → Stress fracture → Complete fracture

Tim Noakes, MD, in *The Lore of Running*, details a four-staged symptomatic progression of stress reaction to stress fracture:

- Stage 1 is characterized by sensations, after running, of vague discomfort poorly localized to the region of the bone injury.
- Stage 2 is characterized by discomfort that is present while running, but may be tolerable enough to "run through."
- Stage 3 is defined as a situation in which the severity of pain prevents running.
- Stage 4 is characterized by the stress reaction having progressed to complete fracture.

Stress fractures are common. Bennell and Brukner (1997) have reported that between 8.3% and 52% of runners cumulatively have histories of stress fracture. The majority of them occur in the lower leg (tibia and fibula) and foot (metatarsals). Although the exact mechanism by which a stress fracture develops is complex and contingent on the multiple interactive mechanisms that we have discussed, there are many well-recognized risks, many of which are avoidable. They are:

1. Low bone density
2. Energy deficit
3. Low calcium diet
4. Female gender
5. Hormonal factors
6. Training errors
7. Biomechanical factors
8. Running mechanics
9. Footwear

For purposes of analysis these factors can be considered individually, but they commonly occur in combination, and it's important to realize that bone injuries often are manifested because of these interactive relationships.

Low Bone Density

It is well established that existing skeletal structural factors contribute to stress fracture risk. The ability of a bone to withstand repetitive low-magnitude loads depends on its mass (how much bone is present) and structure (geometry and shape). As noted by Myburgh and colleagues (1990), low bone density is an etiologic factor for stress fractures in athletes.

Energy Deficit

As we discussed in detail in Chapter 4, energy deficiency may be caused by inadequate dietary intake, excessive energy expenditure through exercise, or a combination of both. Regardless of the cause, energy deficiency leads to changes in bone remodeling, with rate of bone resorption exceeding formation. Repeated bouts of acute or chronic energy deficit leads to an uncoupling of bone remodeling that may be mediated through a number of pathways that include hormones, growth factors, and nutrients. There is robust scientific support for the belief that most bone-related injuries in the athletic population are related to inadequate nutrition and/or energy deficit. For example, in 1995 Bennell and colleagues reported that female athletes with a stress fracture were significantly more likely to have dieted and restricted their food intakes than their non-injured peers.

It is important to realize that although bone injuries generally are seen in runners, the energy-deficit theory of bone injury is especially relevant to those who engage in cross-training or multisport competitors such as duathlon, triathalon, or adventure racing. We encounter many athletes who have had a stable running history, free from bone injuries. However, adding more training hours of non-weight bearing exercise, such as cycling, swimming, or paddling, without a compensatory increase in dietary intake can result in bone injury. Although the fracture is manifested under the mechanical loads of running, it is likely to be the result of the total energy deficit rather than the running per se.

Low Calcium Diet

Dietary calcium intake is inversely related to stress fractures in both males and females. Many individuals who are energy deficient also have insufficient nutrient intake, including calcium. We often encounter stress fractures in endurance athletes who consume less than 600 mg of calcium per day. It is imperative that athletes consume, through diet or supplementation, twice this amount. Whole-food sources of calcium should be the athlete's first choice, as the calcium in real food appears to be absorbed more readily than does the calcium in manufactured food or supplements. In addition, whole foods contain other factors that work synergistically with calcium to improve bone quality. Individuals who are engaged in moderate or heavy training should consider an additional 100–200 mg per day for every hour of exercise beyond their basal calcium requirement (Myburgh, et al., 1988).

Female Athletes

Female athletes are more susceptible to bone injury than males. This is especially true because females have higher rates of eating disorders. Menstrual cycle abnormalities are another important risk factor. Some reports indicate that bone injury or stress fracture is up to 12 times higher in women than men who undergo to the same training program (Brudvig, et al., 1983; Protzman, 1979). The role that gender plays in the development of stress fractures is not well understood, but may be related to several factors, including:

- Higher frequency of disordered eating
- Biomechanical factors including lower extremity alignment
- Smaller bone diameter
- Joint laxity
- Poor muscular strength
- Poor muscular or motor control (neuromuscular considerations)

Hormonal Factors

Multiple studies have reported correlations between low levels of reproductive hormones and bone loss in both males and females. The first clinical challenge is to determine if a stress fracture is related to a hormonal perturbation; the second is to identify the cause of the disturbance. In female athletes, voluntary dietary restraint (disordered eating) is the most likely cause of low estrogen levels. Similar patterns of caloric restriction are seen in male endurance athletes. In such cases, athletes are strongly encouraged to seek assistance from qualified psychological experts who are trained in dealing with such disorders. To rule out hormonally mediated stress fractures, we also recommend a comprehensive screening by a physician with an expertise in exercise endocrinology.

Training Errors

Because a typical bone remodeling cycle requires approximately three months, many bone injuries occur early in a training program. We see many high school track and crosscountry athletes, as well novice adult runners, who develop stress fractures shortly after initiating running. These individuals have little or no understanding of proper running mechanics and do not allow ample time for muscles and bones to adapt to the loading demands of running. Military studies have suggested that the out-of-shape recruit is at greater risk for bone injury (Jones, et al., 1993; Valimaki, et al., 2005; Winfield, et al., 1997). Based on these studies, we recommend that all individuals interested in starting a running program be instructed in proper running mechanics and follow a graduated program under the supervision of a knowledgeable coach or trainer.

In addition to the early stages of new or unsupervised training programs, we see high mileage competitive runners develop bone injuries following a rapid increase in speed work. This problem is much more common in runners who perform the majority of their base mileage with a heel-first landing pattern and then immediately transition to a ball-of-the-foot landing pattern that is consistent with faster running speeds. Because the forces acting on muscles and bones are very different from one style of running to the next, introduction of a different technique is an open invitation for both bone and soft tissue injuries. The likelihood of these injuries can be reduced or prevented by using a consistent running technique through the continuum of running speeds.

Biomechanical Factors

Researchers have learned that stress fractures are more common in individuals with certain anatomic variants, including:

- Leg length discrepancy
- Morton's toe

- High arched rigid (supinated) foot
- Low arched flexible (pronated) foot
- Excessive hip external rotation

Leg length discrepancies may be defined as being either *true* or *apparent*. A true leg length inequality is related to an actual difference in bone length between sides. Either the femur (thigh) or lower leg (tibia) may be shorter on one side resulting in an actual or true inequality. An apparent or functional leg length inequality is said to exist when bone lengths are equal, but another reason exists for one lower extremity functioning in a longer or shorter manner than the other. Common reasons for this functional discrepancy include scoliosis (lateral curve of the spine), flexibility deficit of a muscle (psoas major, iliotibial band), hip abductor weakness, or asymmetry of the inner longitudinal arch of the foot. In 1982 Friberg reported that 87% of army recruits with stress fractures had leg length inequalities. Similarly, in 1996 Bennell and colleagues reported that 70% of track and field athletes diagnosed with stress fracture had a limb length discrepancy.

A complete static and dynamic postural examination that includes standing radiographs, as well as thorough assessment of joint range of motion and soft tissue flexibility, is necessary to determine which type of leg length discrepancy exists. Treatment is then contingent on the nature of the discrepancy. For a true discrepancy, the addition of a shoe lift (internal or external) is most likely indicated. For an apparent discrepancy, a specific program of rehabilitative exercises is necessary to normalize flexibility and/or strength deficits.

Morton's toe is a condition in which the first ray (great toe) is shorter than the second. Clinically, there is a high prevalence of second metatarsal stress fractures in those with a Morton's deformity. Although there is nothing that can be done to alter the actual bone lengths, most individuals with this foot type are found to have compensatory movement patterns that are amenable to treatment. If you have a Morton's foot we recommend an examination by a health care provider with expertise in both running mechanics as well as rehabilitative exercise. Frequently, improvements in ankle dorsiflexion mobility and plantar flexion strength alleviate excessive metatarsal strain.

Individuals with high arches (supinated foot) or low arches (pronated foot) are reportedly at a higher risk for the development of certain stress fractures. Researchers have speculated that extremes of foot posture that are either too rigid or too flexible create circumstances in which abnormal biomechanical forces may precipitate bone injury.

Unfortunately, the studies that have reported such findings have only correlated static measurements of foot posture with injury incidence. What appears to be more relevant is to define how the foot and lower extremity behave dynamically during the running gait.

The degrees of supination and pronation are contingent on other gait factors that are amendable to change with alterations in running technique. As an example, over striding (landing in front of your general center of mass) creates a situation in which landing impact forces as well as the duration of the stance phase are increased. Both of these factors are related to the degree of supination or pronation one exhibits. Therefore, training to bring about alterations in gait can reduce running-related forces as well as moderate abnormal foot mechanics. In our experience, static foot posture is less of a risk for stress fracture development if proper running technique is developed.

Excessive hip external rotation has been cited as a risk factor for tibial stress fracture development. "Excessive" is defined operationally as greater than 60 degrees. The amount of hip rotation can be determined by lying on your back with knees straight and feet pointing directly vertical. Turn your entire lower extremity "outward" so that the lateral border (small toe side) of your foot moves toward the ground. The angle from the starting vertical position to the terminally rotated position is an approximate representation of the degree of hip external rotation. A normal value is 45 degrees. The most common reason for excessive hip external rotation is the geometry or shape of the femur. Clinically, this condition is known as a retroverted hip and is a product of genetics and/or environmental factors during development. Following skeletal maturity, there is no treatment available for decreasing this angle. However, in our experience this finding is less relevant when proper running mechanics are utilized. Specifically, individuals with excessive hip external rotation should not attempt to run with feet facing directly forward, but rather should run with the hip in its own neutral position. For an individual with excessive hip external rotation (and usually a compensatory loss of internal rotation), this will be a slightly externally rotated or toed-out position. This functional mid-range position allows the hip joint and its associated musculature to absorb energy better.

Running Mechanics

Gait mechanics recently have become a focus of scientific inquiry and it is now widely recognized that running mechanics are related to the development of bone injury. In 2006, Milner and colleagues evaluated the gaits of 50 female runners, 25 of whom had a history of a tibial stress fracture (TSF) and 25 of whom had no history of a stress fracture (control group). Because some TSFs are spiral in nature, the free moment (FM) that measures torque around a vertical axis was evaluated. In addition, ground reaction forces, foot placement on the force platform, peak adduction, breaking peak, and impulse were investigated. All variables, with the exception of impulse, were greater in runners with a history of stress fracture. Absolute peak FM had a significant predictive relationship with a history of TSF.

We are not sure why running mechanics have not been considered risk factors before now, but it may be because many people assume that running style is unique to each individual and consequently impossible (or inadvisable) to alter. Conversely, it now is well documented that, with proper instruction, a runner's gait can be modified and that risk factors for bone injury, including impact forces and time on support, can be decreased.

In 2004 Nicholas Romanov and his colleagues, working in the laboratory of Dr. Tim Noakes, instructed 20 heel-toe runners in the Pose Method of running. The performed gait analysis before and after 7.5 hours of training over five consecutive days. They found that as a result of the training knee power absorption (W/kg) was significantly reduced (7.01 +/– 1.75 vs. 3.70 +/– 1.40). In another study, honors student Hannah Zoller (2008), working under the direction of Dr. John Challis at The Pennsylvania State University, evaluated the biomechanical forces of seven heel-toe runners before and after they received three hours of Pose Method running training. Results demonstrated a significant reduction in peak hip resultant joint moment (Nm) (247.1 +/– 58.0 vs. 72.1 +/– 48.2) after training.

The tenets of Pose style running as described by Nicholas Romanov include:

- Ball-of-the-foot landing
- Vertical alignment of ankle, hip, and shoulder during stance
- Emphasis on high cadence (>90 per minute)
- Maximal use of elastic return versus muscular energy
- Maintenance of a flexed knee throughout gait
- Maximal use of gravity for horizontal movement

Interested readers may consult with Dr. Nicholas Romanov (posetech.com) or one of his certified running coaches for information regarding the Pose Method of running and opportunities to receive training. In particular, we endorse the following coaches with whom we have had the opportunity to collaborate: Jack Becker (TX), Michael Collins (CA), Lynn McFadden (FL), Connie Sol (FL), Joe Sparks (OH), Josh Gold (NY), and Martha Michael (PA).

Friend and respected running coach Jack Becker provided the following perspective on his personal training philosophy

> I approach my Training with an emphasis on the T, a duality; T for technique and T for training. The technical aspect is always my primary focus with conditioning a natural outcome of correct movement. With well-executed technique, I am able to run more volume and as often described more quality runs; although, personally, I believe every run is of benefit, quality. Along with volume, I can also run with intensity more often due to less chance of undue soreness, potential injury, and faster recovery. I base this on comparison with training periods without a concentration on technique and using a heel/toe running pattern.

When asked about performance limitations, he told us,

> My limiters to a focus on technique are fatigue and loss of concentration. These are normal and, generally, fatigue can easily lead to a loss of concentration, but can be separate limiters. Running with volume, intensity or both will generate fatigue if either or both are maintained for long enough. If this happens, and I have not met my goal for the session, I do not automatically suspend the run. If I can drop pace to a level that I can maintain technique, I will continue to run. With the Pose Method, I can reduce the perception of lean and range of motion while maintaining cadence. If I get to a point that, I cannot hold technique, I will stop and walk, recover and make a decision to continue or save it for another day.

Jack began his marathon running career in January 2002 at the age of 56. His best marathon finishing time to date is 3:22, which he accomplished at the St. George Marathon in Utah. He believes his best race performance was a 3:25 Boston Marathon finish in 2006.

Footwear

Traditional studies have found no significant relationship between footwear and stress fracture. However, now some people believe that the modern running shoe plays a causal rather than a protective role in overuse injuries, including stress fracture. Shoes with substantial heel counters, motion control systems, and cushioning could increase injury risk for several reasons, including:

- Gait alteration
- Reduced intrinsic impact-moderating behavior
- Intrinsic foot weakness
- Perceptual deficits

Our observations of the running gaits of nearly all distance runners wearing modern running shoes reveals a heel-first landing pattern. Conversely, with no education or suggestion to change, when these runners are asked to run without their shoes, most automatically increase the degree of knee flexion and land on the balls of their feet. Both of these modifications result in significantly less impact to bones and joints. Gordon Pirie, a former world record holder and Olympic medal winner, wrote in *Running Fast and Injury Free* (see Gilbody, 2002, Chapter Two, "Why Athletes Fail"),

> The prevailing attitude amongst runners and those who coach or advise them, it that a failure to attain specific goals is the result of either bad luck, lack of talent, or some form of psychological shortcoming on the part of the athlete. Usually, none of these reasons is true. Athletes fail so often because they are not trained to succeed. Most athletes employ training methods or have lifestyles which make it possible for them to perform up to their expectations and aspirations. Another important factor is the poor design of most running shoes.

When a runner places his or her foot in a shoe with an extensive arch support or adds an orthotic insert, the intrinsic foot muscles and inner longitudinal arch are not required to be activated to the degree that they are when running barefoot or in a minimalist shoe. Consequences include limitations in mobility (especially the heel cord) and strength. Mobility loss combined with intrinsic muscular weakness and poor fatigue resistance render the foot and lower leg more susceptible to injury. Researchers Rao and Joseph (1992) examined 2,300 children between the ages of four and 13 and found that the flat feet was more than three times more likely in those children who wore shoes than those who did not. They concluded that wearing shoes during early childhood development is detrimental to the development of a normal arch.

Although many in the medical community do not consider the process to be tenable, it is possible to strengthen the weakened muscles and improve arch integrity in adults who have a history of extensive shoe wear. In a very enlightening study by Robbins and Hannah (1987), 17 normally shod recreational runners were instructed to increase barefoot activity gradually over several weeks and to maintain this activity for approximately four months. Each runner's feet were evaluated for structural changes at regular intervals. Results showed significant improvement in the anatomical structure and function of the arch.

The sole of the foot is richly endowed with nerve endings, the purpose of which is to provide the brain (central nervous system) with nearly instant information regarding the surface on which you are standing (or running). This afferent information allows the brain to orchestrate the appropriate motor or efferent neurologic messages back to the muscles of the lower extremity in order to best shield our bones as well as to adapt to the infinite intricacies of the ground. Modern footwear, with its extensive cushioning, effectively eliminates the sensory information that is normally relayed to the brain. As a result, the protection of our skeleton by muscle contraction is reduced.

For instance, Robbins and Waked (1997) found that as the amount of padding in a running shoe increases, ground reaction force increases. In another compelling study by researchers from Rush Medical College in Chicago (Shakoor and Block, 2006), 75 study participants with knee osteoarthritis were evaluated while walking in their everyday walking shoes and in the barefoot condition. The results demonstrated that the peak joint loads at the hips and knees decreased significantly during barefoot walking, with a 11.9% reduction noted in the knee adduction moment (in this context, adduction refers to a collapse of the knee toward midline). Stride, cadence, and range of motion at the lower extremity joints also changed significantly, but these changes could not explain the reduction in peak joint loads. The researchers concluded that shoes may detrimentally increase loads on the lower extremity joints and that modern shoe design may need to be reevaluated.

In order to promote improved foot strength and sensitivity we recommend the following:

- Gradually increase the amount of time you spend wearing no shoes.
- Consider switching your everyday footwear to a minimalist style shoe that has a thin, flexible sole without an arch support or elevated heel.
- Perform strengthening exercises for the muscles of the lower leg and foot that support the inner longitudinal arch.
- Gradually transition to a lightweight running shoe that provides less stability and cushion.

Although there has been a surge of public interest in barefoot running, in part as a result of Christopher McDougall's best selling book *Born to Run,* we have treated a number of runners with stress-related soft tissue and bone injuries as a direct result of attempting too much too soon. The results of the Robbins and Hannah study are especially important to consider. Increase in arch height that was observed in their study, presumably related to improved intrinsic foot strength, required approximately three months to achieve. This is an important time frame as it parallels the time required for one bone remodeling cycle to occur. This duration may be a reasonable generic recommendation for the length of time necessary to transition from a supportive to a minimalist shoe or to the barefoot condition. That said, there simply is not a-one-size-fits-all approach.

To illustrate this point we will consider two examples. Recently one of us (TJW) had the opportunity to work with two recreational triathletes who had very different barefoot running experiences. The first, a male, is a top-notch endurance athlete. He had competed very successfully in ironman triathlon, marathon, and ultramarathon running. Unfortunately, he developed a case of heel pain that had prevented him from running for three months. My examination revealed a loss of ankle mobility, which responded well to a program of self-treatment exercise and manipulation. Following three treatment sessions he was able to return to running. In an attempt to reduce the likelihood of the condition returning, I recommended that he modify his running mechanics and suggested a minimalist running shoe with less material under the heel. Within six weeks time he was able to run continuously for up to 2.5 hours with no complications.

In comparison, a female recreational triathlete of similar age came to the clinic with a history of metatarsal stress fracture that began after she attempted to run with no shoes for less than 15 minutes. Following a six-week recovery period, during which she was placed in an ankle/foot immobilizer, she attempted to return to running in a minimalist shoe and developed a subsequent fracture of a cuboid that required an additional six weeks recovery time. Hormonal and bone density testing revealed a normal hormone profile with slightly lower than average bone mineral density for her age. This patient's energy and calcium intakes were marginally low. Because of her skeleton's apparent fragility we recommended refraining from running for six months to allow for long-term structural adaptations in the foot to occur as well as to improve that daily energy and calcium intake.

If you are an adult who has become accustomed to wearing a rigid shoe with an elevated heel for daily use as well as a motion control or stability shoe for running, your intrinsic foot musculature and connective tissues may be in a deconditioned state. If that is the case, it is important to make changes gradually and to remember that improvements in these tissues will require several months to be fully realized. There may also be a significant advantage to consulting a medical professional (physician, podiatrist, physical therapist) with specialized training in rehabilitation of the foot as there are many specific exercises that may complement your self-treatment.

Summary

Stress fractures are defined as being microscopic traumatic injuries to bone in which the rate of bone damage exceeds the rate at which it can be remodeled. The cause of a stress fracture may be related to a multitude of well-defined factors that by convention are described as being intrinsic or extrinsic.

Injuries to bone exist on a continuum: the more mild are defined as a stress reaction and the more severe are diagnosed as a fracture. The rate at which a stress fracture heals is variable, but in general the prognosis for recovery is good. Reducing the likelihood of a recurrence is contingent on the identification of the original cause. Clinical experience shows that the most common causal factors are low bone mass, energy deficit, low calcium diet, running mechanics, and footwear.

REFERENCES

Arendse R, Noakes T, Azevedo L, Romanov N, Schwellnus M, Fletcher G (2004) Reduced eccentric loading of the knee with the Pose running method. *Medicine & Science in Sports and Exercise* 36(2):272–277.

Bennell K, Brukner P (1997) Epidemiology and site specificity of stress fractures. *Clinical Sports Medicine* 16:179–196.

Bennell K, Malcolm S, Thomas S, Ebeling P, McCrory P, Wark J, Brukner P (1995) Risk factors for stress fractures in female track-and-field athletes: a retrospective analysis. *Clinical Journal of Sport Medicine* 5:229–235.

Bennell K, Malcolm S, Thomas S (1996) Risk factors for stress fractures in track and field athletes: a twelve-month prospective study. *American Journal of Sports Medicine* 24(6):810–818.

Brudvig T, Grudger T, Obermeyer L (1983) Stress fractures in 295 trainees: a one year study of incidence as related to age, sex, and race. *Military Medicine* 148:666–667.

Friberg O (1982) Leg length asymmetry in stress fractures: a clinical and radiological study. *Journal of Sports Medicine and Physical Fitness* 22:485–488.

Jones BH, Bovee MW, Harris JM, Cowan DN (1993) Intrinsic risk factors for exercise-related injuries among male and female army trainees. *American Journal of Sports Medicine* 21:705–710.

McDougall Christopher (2009) *Born to Run.* New York and Canada: Alfred A. Knopf division of Random House, Inc.

Milner C, Davis I, Hamill J (2006) Free moment as a predictor of tibial stress fracture in distance runners. *Journal of Biomechanics* 39(15):2819–2825.

Myburgh K, Grobler N, Noakes T (1988) Factors associated with shin soreness in athletes. *Physician and Sportsmedicine* 16:129–134.

Myburgh K, Hutchins J, Fataar A, Hough S, Noakes T (1990) Low bone density is an etiologic factor for stress fractures in athletes. *Annals of Internal Medicine* 113:754–759.

Noakes T (2003) *The Lore of Running,* 4th edition. Champaign, IL: Human Kinetics Publishing.

Pirie G (No date). *Running Fast and Injury Free.* Full text copy edited by John Gilbody, www.gordonpirie.com.

Protzman R (1979) Physiologic performance of women compared to men: observations of cadets at the United States Military Academy. *American Journal of Sports Medicine* 7:191–194.

Rao U, Joseph B (1992) The influence of footwear on the prevalence of flat foot, a survey of 2300 children. *The Journal of Bone and Joint Surgery* 74B (4):525–527.

Robbins S, Hanna A (1987) Running related injury prevention through barefoot adaptations. *Medicine and Science in Sports and Exercise* 19(2):148–156.

Robbins S, Waked E (1997) Foot position awareness: the effect of footwear on instability, excessive impact, and ankle spraining. *Critical Reviews in Physical and Rehabilitative Medicine* 9(1):53–74.

Shakoor N, Block JA (2006) Walking barefoot decreases loading on the lower extremity joints in knee osteoarthritis. *Arthritis and Rheumatism* 54(9):2923–2927.

Valimaki V, Alfthan H, Lehmuskallio E (2005) Risk factors for clinical stress fractures in male military recruits: a prospective cohort study. *Bone* 37(2):267–273.

Winfield A, Moore J, Bracker M (1997) Risk factors associated with stress reactions in female marines. *Military Medicine* 162:698–702.

Zoller H (2008) Ground Reaction Forces and Joint Moments in Pose Running. Unpublished undergraduate thesis, The Pennsylvania State University. Department of Kinesiology and Schreyer Honors College.

CHAPTER FOURTEEN

Rehabilitation of Stress Fractures

When considering the rehabilitation of a stress fracture, one must first understand why the injury occurred in the first place. Stress fractures generally are the culmination of several risk factors that were outlined in the Chapter 13. Once these factors can be identified, their elimination must become a cornerstone of treatment so the problem does not recur. In our experience, the most common elements that need to be addressed are poor running technique, poor nutrition, and low bone mass.

Poor running technique is defined by a heel strike landing pattern that occurs in front of the general center of mass. This results in significant "braking" or eccentric loading of the lower extremities as well as prolonged time spent in the stance phase of running. Additionally, many runners do not realize that when running technique is faltering, as in the latter stages of a marathon, injury risk is elevated. Consequently, it is critical to educate runners not only in proper technique but also in perceiving and understanding good versus faulty form.

Chronic energy deficit is defined by inadequate dietary intake, excessive energy expenditure, or a combination of both. It should be determined if the energy deficit is the result of a purposeful imbalance, as in dieting or anorexia, or instead due to simple neglect. If disordered eating behavior is involved, referral to a mental health specialist with a background in treating the endurance athlete is paramount, since early intervention is associated with better outcomes.

Reproductive hormone imbalance is a very common finding in stress-fractured endurance athletes. Frequently the problem can be attributed to the emotional and physical stress of heavy training or competition in conjunction with poor diet and inadequate recovery. If an athlete provides a history of overtraining symptoms or relentless fatigue, a complete physical examination that includes hormone testing by a primary care sports medicine physician is advisable.

Unfortunately, many endurance athletes are unaware that they have developed low bone mass. It is not until they experience a stress fracture that diagnostic testing is performed, which then indicates the extent to which their bone mass already has been compromised. Because bone loss is easier to prevent than it is to restore, the rehabilitation and long-term management of an athlete with established osteoporosis is challenging.

Establishing a Diagnosis

The diagnosis of a stress reaction or fracture is clinically straightforward for those medical professionals who are familiar with such injuries. Many athletes will report a period of time during which symptoms were mild and of only nuisance quality. Then, if training continues and injury severity increases, they report that additional running became impossible because of severe pain. The inability to run is what ultimately forces athletes to seek treatment. Often recovery time can be reduced if an athlete seeks treatment early.

In many circumstances, the early recognition of a stress injury to bone may enable an athlete to continue to run, albeit in a modified manner. For example, we often treat runners who began to experience lower leg (shin) pain when they added speed or track workouts. Many of them can continue to run if their technique is improved and/or their program is simply modified to avoid speed-training sessions until symptoms subside.

If an injury is allowed to progress to the point at which running even with proper technique is impossible, more aggressive treatment is needed. For an athlete who is comfortable walking, all that is necessary is to avoid running long enough for the fracture to heal. During this time it is important to start an alternative form of exercise in order to prevent fitness losses as well as to minimize the depressive affect that often accompanies an injury and the absence of exercise. Pool running is an excellent option; other options include a stationary bike trainer, crosscountry ski simulator, rowing ergometer, or elliptical trainer. One study (Eyestone, et al., 1993) showed that six weeks of running in a pool with a floatation device maintained VO2 max and two-mile running performance of trained athletes just as effectively as did an equivalent land-based program.

Strength exercises for the body parts that are not injured also should be encouraged. Because stress fractures generally are sensitive to forces that produce strain (bending), longitudinal compression loading involving the fractured bone generally is tolerated well at this stage. Many athletes with stress fractures of the lower leg (tibia or fibula) can perform general strengthening exercises, including deadlifts, squats, and rows, with no increase in pain.

The early stage of rehabilitation is an excellent time to dedicate to reducing strength deficits or mobility impairments identified by a medical professional. Alternatively, some athletes will benefit from a complete respite from exercise. In select cases, a complete departure from exercise can produce more thorough physical and emotional rejuvenation. This is the case for athletes who have been suffering from symptoms of chronic fatigue, depression, or overtraining.

In cases in which even walking has become painful, a reduction in loading with the use of crutches or an immobilization device (removable cast or brace) is indicated. Such unloading measures provide an environment that is conducive for healing and also prevent collateral damage to other body parts that are subjected to the abnormal loads that accompany a limp. If reduced weight bearing or immobilization is necessary, all attempts should be made to maintain normal range of motion and strength of the involved joints and soft tissues through specific exercises that are recommended by your medical team.

We recommend the least amount of unloading or immobilization necessary to provide a pain-free walking gait. Complete immobilization (casting) or non-weight bearing gait patterns should be avoided if possible. These extreme measures commonly induce stiffness, weakness, and loss of bone mineral. As one example of the case for maintaining bone loading during treatment, Swenson and colleagues (1997) reported that athletes treated with pneumatic leg braces returned to full, unrestricted activity within three weeks, whereas athletes who were treated in a more conventional manner required 13 weeks to recover from tibial stress fractures.

The amount of time required for a stress fracture to heal is contingent on its location and severity. Most stress fractures heal in about four to 16 weeks. Injuries to small bones (metatarsals) heal significantly faster than large bones (femur or pelvis). Injuries that are confined to the superficial aspects of a bone (cortex) resolve more quickly than do those that have advanced through the cortex and involve the deeper (intramedullary) regions of bone.

Diagnostic Studies

Because the diagnosis of a stress injury to bone generally is made on clinical grounds, diagnostic studies such as plain radiographs (x-rays) are considered ancillary rather than necessary. This is because the high incidence of a false-negative result is elevated for three weeks following injury. Only after the fracture begins to unite does any radiographic evidence of the injury become evident. Until a certain diagnosis is made, it is prudent to treat the injury as if it were a stress fracture, with activity reduced to the level at which pain is eliminated. Most physicians now rely on either the magnetic resonance image (MRI) or bone scan to confirm the suspected diagnosis of a stress fracture. Both of these diagnostic techniques are sensitive and specific for the presence of a bone injury (stress reaction or stress fracture).

MRI is considered to be the gold standard for the diagnosis of stress fracture. It is capable of providing detailed images of bones in any plane as well as defining areas of swelling and inflammation. Unlike traditional radiographs, MRI uses no ionizing radiation, instead generating a magnetic field to align the nuclear magnetization of hydrogen atoms in body water. Radiofrequency fields are used to alter the alignment of this magnetization, causing the hydrogen nuclei to produce a rotating magnetic field detectable by the scanner. The signal is manipulated by other magnetic fields to construct a detailed image of the bony architecture. A standard MRI requires less than an hour to complete. Since there is no physical contact or manipulation of the injury site, the test is completely painless. The MRI does produce a loud knocking sound, but this may be blunted partially by the use of ear protectors or headphones that allow the patient to listen to music. The patient must remain motionless for the duration of the procedure.

Bone scans also can be used to detect abnormalities that are not apparent on standard radiographs. A small amount of radioactive medicine is injected with a needle and syringe. After ample time for the medication to circulate and infiltrate the skeleton, the body is scanned with a gamma camera that is sensitive to the radiation emitted from the injected medication. The amount of medicine that collects in the bones is related to the degree of metabolic activity or turnover. Regions of bone that have been injured are very active metabolically and therefore attract a heavy concentration of the radioactive medicine. The actual scanning process is painless but requires the patient to remain still for the duration of the test. Bone scans can be performed of the entire body or any selected region (lower leg, foot) and in either a single or phased manner.

It is interesting to note that many runners have regions of increased uptake or "hot spots" that appear on a bone scan that are not symptomatic. Such lesions most likely represent stress reactions (pre-stress fractures) that are not significant enough to cause pain or functional limitation. A study by Zwas and colleagues illustrates this point (1987). They performed bone scans on 310 military recruits suspected of having stress fractures. In 235 patients, 391 stress fractures were diagnosed. Forty percent of the lesions were asymptomatic. Most of the lesions were in the tibia (72%); 87% of the subjects had one or two lesions; and 13% had three to five lesions.

Recovery following most stress fractures follows a predictable and successful course. However, there are several points that must be considered during rehabilitation. Long-term success is contingent on:

- The abolition of pain and/or swelling
- Recovery of normal range of motion in all joints that influence the fracture site
- Recovery of normal flexibility (muscle length)
- Recovery of normal movement quality (neuromuscular control)
- Recovery of normal strength
- Recovery of normal balance
- Recovery of normal elasticity
- Development and proficiency of proper running technique
- Recovery of mental confidence and loss of fear

Rehabilitation of athletes who have sustained stress fractures must be individualized and based on their unique training history, age, health status, bone quality, nutritional state, hormonal status, and performance level. The rate at which a healthy, 22-year-old male, division-I college crosscountry athlete progresses to running 60 miles per week may be quite different than the rate at which a 56-year-old female breast cancer survivor with a chronic history of estrogen deficiency returns to running 25 miles per week. Let's consider these two cases in detail.

Case Study 1
A 22-year-old male collegiate crosscountry and track athlete reported to his team physician with complaints of right lower leg pain in January 2007. He had first noticed the symptoms within the first two weeks of the winter indoor track season and pain had increased to the point that running was not possible. Physical evaluation revealed that he was generally healthy and had localized tenderness and swelling

over the anterior medial tibia. He had no significant pain with walking but the "hop test" showed that pain prevented him from hopping on the injured side. His medical systems and nutritional screening was normal. His medical history revealed that he had a mild ankle sprain on the same side during the last meet of the fall crosscountry season (approximately five weeks prior). MRI revealed the presence of a mild stress fracture on the cortex (surface) of the tibia.

Because the patient had no pain with walking, the physician did not recommend crutches or bracing. He was directed to refrain from team practices and to report to the university physical therapy department to initiate rehabilitation.

The rehabilitation plan was influenced by the discovery during physical evaluation of a 1.5 cm leg length inequality in which the stress-fractured side was shorter than the uninvolved side. Additionally, a 10 degree loss of ankle joint mobility and a 20% reduction in calf strength were identified on the side of the stress fracture. The patient reported that following his ankle sprain five weeks ago, the ankle had felt stiff and weak.

It was hypothesized that because of the leg length inequality as well as the loss of ankle mobility and strength, abnormal forces were transmitted to the tibia during running, resulting in a stress fracture of the tibia. Treatment goals included the following:

1. Maintain general fitness with alternative exercise
2. Balance lower extremity leg lengths with the use of a shoe insert
3. Restore normal ankle joint mobility and strength
4. Increase level of loading in a progressive pain free manner
5. Return the patient to team practice/competition

During treatment week number one a 0.75 cm shoe insert was fabricated, designed to reduce 50% of his leg length asymmetry. For many individuals with long-standing leg length inequalities, starting with an insert that reduces the deficit by 30–50% is prudent. Rehabilitation exercises designed to normalize ankle mobility and strength also were initiated at this time. Overall fitness was maintained with 45 minutes of pool running performed twice daily, a regime which closely matched his current volume of training. He continued to perform general strength exercises for the upper body, trunk, and hips with his teammates twice per week.

By week number two it was clear that the patient had no difficulty accommodating to the shoe lift. In fact, he reported that the lift seemed to reduce lower back pain that he had previously experienced with periods of prolonged standing. Ankle joint mobility now was normal relative to the uninvolved side, but ankle strength remained deficient. Palpation revealed that there was no longer any detectable swelling, but residual tenderness persisted. Treatment consisted of exercises to maintain range of motion, along with a continuation of specific strengthening exercises for the muscles of the lower leg and foot. General conditioning was modified to include a 60-minute session of pool running in the morning and a 30-minute session of fast walking in the afternoon on the university's indoor track with the patient wearing his customary running shoes (spikeless racing flats) with the shoe insert in place. Additionally, pre-running technique drills that involved no jumping or landing were initiated.

Treatment week three demonstrated that swelling and tenderness was fully resolved. Strength testing showed normal results relative to the uninvolved side. We requested that the patient continue with the morning pool running sessions but reduce their duration to 45 minutes. The afternoon session was to include 30 minutes of track walking followed by 10–15 minutes of barefooted walking and balance drills to be performed in the sand (long-jump pit). Strength levels appeared grossly intact, but single-leg standing balance appeared slightly decreased versus the uninvolved side. Sand walking or running is an excellent way to improve intrinsic foot strength and fatigue resistance and serves as an unstable base for balance exercises.

Treatment week number four remained the same as week number three, but three sessions of sand walking were replaced with light *plyometric exercises* in order to restore the athlete's elasticity and gradually to increase the forces through the lower extremities. In Mark Albert's book *Eccentric Muscle Training in Sports and Orthopaedics* (1995) plyometric exercise is defined as "a quick powerful movement involving a prestretching or counter movement that activates the stretch-shortening cycle." The most easily recognized example of a stretch-shortening cycle is a standard reflex test in which the shortening of a muscle (the knee "jerk") is induced by tapping (stretching) a tendon with a reflex hammer. The phenomenon is related to complex interactions between the body's nervous system and mechanical (viscoelastic) properties of muscles and dense connective tissues (tendons).

When muscles and tendons are stretched quickly, specialized receptors (muscle spindles and golgi tendon organs) provide feedback to the central nervous system. This afferent information influences resting muscle tone, kinesthetic awareness, and the performance of certain motor patterns. The ability to effectively harness stored elastic energy is affected by several variables including both the magnitude and the velocity of the applied stretch. The most important consideration is that the stretch be applied in a short, quick manner.

Please note that plyometric exercises are not yielding or eccentric exercises. Often there is confusion among trainers and athletes alike regarding the difference between these two exercise modes. Examples of an eccentric or yielding action would be "sticking" a landing during a gymnastics dismount during which the energy of the landing is absorbed by flexion of the legs. The prolonged nature of this eccentric muscle action effectively dampens rather than facilitates the reversal of movement. Plyometric exercises should be considered elastic or bouncing in nature. The most important element to consider when teaching or performing elastic exercises is to minimize the time between the stretch and shortening phases. This transitional phase between movement directions is known as the amortization phase and can be defined as "the electromechanical delay between eccentric and concentric contraction during which the muscle must switch from overcoming work to imparting the necessary amount of acceleration in the required direction" (Albert, 1995, pp. 64–65).

We often utilize small amplitude plyometric exercises in the clinic both as a means to assess a patient's neuromuscular control (and fatigue resistance) as well as a way to recondition tissues and improve performance. Examples of safe plyometric exercises include "bouncing" in place (quick bounces on the balls of the feet), jumping jacks (traditional, diagonal, forward/backward), rope skipping, and tuck jumps.

During treatment week number five, running was introduced during the afternoon session. After a light active warm up consisting of running drills and plyometrics, the athlete's running technique was evaluated and determined to be satisfactory. He was requested to run 4 × 400 meters with a two minute walking recovery between running intervals. The intensity of running was 3–4/10 scale that corresponded to a light or moderate effort. We emphasized the need for perfect technique and encouraged him to remain balanced and relaxed while maintaining a feeling of lightness on his feet. If pain increased in intensity, exercise was to be stopped. He was asked to perform between four and eight running intervals of variable distances (between 200–800) per day over the next week in order to provide a loading stimulus to the injury site as well as restore mind-body awareness and improve confidence. Total running time was approximately 12 minutes.

Treatment weeks six through eight consisted of gradually increasing the athlete's total running time to approximately 20–24 minutes per day. We continued to use a variable distance interval format on the indoor track, as this is the surface on which the athlete trains and competes during the winter season. The direction in which the athlete ran on the track was alternated in order to load the lower extremities in a symmetrical manner. The athlete continued to deny experiencing any pain and there was no increase in tenderness or signs of swelling following his running sessions.

Treatment week nine included a return to formal team practices. The athlete's coaches were helpful in allowing him to transition back to full participation over the next three weeks at which time he successfully participated in his first indoor meet.

The patient in this case study was able to advance his running volume and intensity relatively rapidly because it appeared that his injury was most likely a consequence of the deficits induced by a recent ankle sprain and perhaps also to a true leg length inequality. The patient had no other risk factors, excellent running technique, and several years of consistent and uninterrupted running.

Case Study 2
A 56-year-old female breast cancer survivor with a history of recurrent stress fractures was referred to physical therapy in the spring of 2006. She had been diagnosed with breast cancer in 2002 and underwent treatment that included radical mastectomy and chemotherapy. Following her cancer treatment she had made significant lifestyle changes that included regular exercise and a low fat diet in attempt to lose weight. Her weight loss regime consisted of daily walking and a high-carbohydrate diet. Total weight loss was approximately 35 pounds between 2003 and 2005. As the patient's fitness level improved she started to integrate running into her exercise program. As a result she developed a stress fracture of the calcaneus (heel) on the right side in the spring of 2005 and two metatarsal stress fractures on the left in the fall of 2005. Because of her recurrent injuries she requested that her primary care physician refer her to our clinic in hopes of helping her return to recreational running. Her long-term goal was to resume running 25 miles per week.

Evaluation of the patient in May 2006 revealed normal lower extremity alignment in the standing position with the exception of a mildly flattened inner longitudinal arch, slightly more pronounced on the left side. Observation of her walking gait demonstrated that her knees collapsed toward the midline (adduction) during the stance phase. This appeared to be related to intrinsic foot weakness as well as weakness of the hip abductor muscles (muscles on the outside of the hip). Analysis of running gait demonstrated a heel-first landing pattern with slow cadence. Typical running speed was 10-plus minutes per mile and cadence was approximately 78–80 foot strikes per minute (recorded as foot strikes per minute on one side). At the time of evaluation the patient was walking every day for between 30 and 60 minutes. She wore a stability type running shoe with extensive arch support and heel counter. The shoe was advertised as a model suited to individuals with excessive pronation. The patient had not run since the fall of 2005, at which time she had been placed in an ankle immobilizing brace for six weeks secondary to her metatarsal stress fractures. DEXA scan results demonstrated that her current level of bone mass was low; she was diagnosed with osteoporosis at the lumbar spine and hip and osteopenia at the forearm. She expressed a great fear of returning to running because of her past experience of multiple fractures.

Treatment goals included:

1. Improve trunk (spine, pelvis) and lower extremity muscular strength in order to reduce or reverse bone loss.
2. Improve muscular strength of the foot and reduce the collapse of the inner longitudinal arch.
3. Ensure adequate dietary protein, fat, and calcium intake to maximize muscular and skeletal adaptations to exercise.
4. Improve running technique:
    a. Eliminate over striding/heel strike landing
    b. Reduce knee adduction (collapse of knee toward midline)
    c. Increase cadence rate
5. Return to recreational running with no additional fractures.

Initial treatment recommendations consisted of instruction in a home-based exercise program to improve muscular strength and foot posture. These exercises included body weight exercises, since balance and control were insufficient to be considered safe to utilize externally applied loads. These exercises included balance training (single-leg support on an inflatable disc), single and double legged squats, and abdominal exercises (Janda sit-ups). Particular emphasis was placed on improving stability of the trunk and lower extremity with alignment of the lower extremities in neutral. Additionally, the patient was asked to avoid wearing shoes for one hour per day while in her home (since she had sustained her metatarsal stress fractures she refrained from walking without shoe support). The patient lived a great distance from the clinic so it was agreed that she would return for follow up in one month. Additionally, it was suggested that she meet with a registered dietician for advice regarding the adequacy of her diet.

When the patient returned for follow up she demonstrated a significant increase in hip strength and slight improvement in foot posture. She had increased calcium intake to 1,200 mg per day and protein intake to approximately 100 g per day. Additionally, she increased dietary fat to 30% and decreased carbohydrate intake to maintain caloric balance. Prior to meeting with the dietician, protein intake had been 65 g/day, calcium intake less than 600 mg/day, and the percentage of daily calories from fat 10%. Treatment included an upgrade of her home strengthening program that included the addition of resistance exercises and the suggestion that she acquire a pair of flat (no heel) shoes with minimal or no arch support or stability for everyday activities. She would continue to wear her stability shoes for standing or walking for prolonged periods. The patient was encouraged to discontinue wearing shoes altogether while she was in her home. She was to return in one month, at which time we planned on initiating running specific drills.

In July the patient returned, very pleased with her progress. She was well aware that her overall level of strength had improved: she now could ascend stairs with heavy loads (groceries and laundry) much more easily and noted that the alignment of her foot/ankle was less collapsed. Treatment during this visit included initiation of running specific drills with an emphasis on reducing her over striding tendency and improving her cadence. Our goal was to have her land directly below rather than in front of her center of mass and to increase cadence to over 90 foot strikes per minute. We recommended that she practice the running drills daily and continue with her walking routine. Additionally, we suggested that she obtain a lightweight running shoe with no significant arch support or heel counter for her daily walks. She was invited to return in one month, at which time we planned on evaluating her running form and advancing her running based on her skill level.

In August the patient returned to the clinic anxious about the possibility of returning to running. Examination of her foot posture revealed essentially normal foot/ankle alignment with no collapse of her arch. She related that she was having no foot or lower leg discomfort during or following her daily walks in her minimalist shoe. Examination of her running technique revealed that she started her running with excellent form but that it quickly degraded after only 30 meters as she started to increase her lower extremity range of motion. As a result, her landing pattern was too far in front of her center of mass (over striding). She was perceptive enough to detect this difference and we attempted to extend the duration of her quality running technique through drills as well as with the use of an EZ running belt, an excellent training aid that was developed by running coach and trainer Joe Sparks (fitnesswithjoe.com).

Because this patient sensed when her running form started to deteriorate, we suggested that she integrate short running intervals into her daily walking program. The length of the intervals was to be determined by the length of time for which she could maintain quality running technique. She was to return in six weeks.

Upon her return in late September she was far more comfortable with her new running form and was performing a daily walk-run interval session lasting approximately 60 minutes per day. Over the course of the past six weeks, the total amount of running time had been increased from 10 to approximately 25 minutes per day. She felt competent running on flat surfaces and running uphill but had difficulties maintaining form while running downhill. With this in mind, the treatment session was directed at improving her skill level during downhill running. By the end of this session she appeared to have an improved capacity for adjusting her technique to a variety of downhill grades and was discharged from formal care with the recommendation that she return in the future on an as-needed basis.

The patient in this case study was advanced through a treatment program very slowly because she had several risk factors for stress fracture. These included low bone mass, a history of estrogen deficiency, poor diet, lower-extremity weakness, and poor running technique. Her rehabilitation required five physical therapy treatment sessions over six months.

Medical Management

Additional treatment modalities that may complement rehabilitation include pharmacologic agents or electrical and electromagnetic fields. Nonsteroidal anti-inflammatory drugs (NSAID) are frequently prescribed to athletes for sports-related overuse injuries. They commonly are administered for their analgesic and anti-inflammatory properties. The effects of NSAIDs have been studied extensively in animal models and the majority of the research indicates a detrimental effect on fracture healing (Allen, et al., 1980; Altman, et al., 1995).

Current research in humans offers no firm evidence regarding the use of NSAIDs and stress fracture management. However, some studies suggest that NSAID use may be detrimental to the healing rate of other fracture types or surgical fusions using bone grafts (Adolphson, et al., 1993; Reuben and Ekman, 2005; Reuben, et al.,

2005). Given these concerns, individuals with bone injuries should refrain from taking any more of these medications than is absolutely necessary for pain control during the acute phase of rehabilitation.

The bisphosphonates comprise a class of drugs that have been used to treat a variety of bone disorders, including osteoporosis. They act directly on the osteoclast to inhibit bone resorption. There has been some interest among researchers in studying their effect on fractures. From a theoretical standpoint, if bone resorption were decreased while bone formation processes were maintained, there could be a prophylactic value in their administration to high-risk athletes. However, although there have been some studies of their use in treatment (Milgrom, et al., 2004), to date none have demonstrated any value for stress fracture prevention.

Stewart and colleagues (2005) reported that they successfully administered pamidronate, a second-generation biphosphonate, to five female collegiate athletes with tibial stress fractures. A 30 mg dose was given intravenously over two hours, followed by four additional weekly treatments in 60 mg or 90 mg doses. Four of the five subjects were reported to be able to continue training with no time lost, while the fifth patient missed only three weeks of training. At a minimum of 49 months follow-up, all of these athletes remained asymptomatic.

Parathyroid hormone (PTH) conserves body calcium and has an anabolic effect on bone. However, in high doses it may result in bone resorption. In 2002, the United States Food and Drug Administration approved teriparatide, a synthetic form of PTH, for the treatment of osteoporosis. It has been speculated that PTH could play a role in the treatment of resistant stress fractures. To date, there have been no well-controlled clinical studies to validate its use in human stress fractures, although earlier results of animal studies have been favorable (Holzer, et al., 1999; Blick, et al., 2008).

Calcium and vitamin D intake are critical for bone health, and their supplemental use during fracture healing has been established in animal and human studies. However, no well-controlled studies have determined the optimal supplemental doses to use during the rehabilitation of a stress fracture. Most of the studies have compared experimental groups taking recommended levels of calcium and vitamin D to control groups of subjects who are calcium and vitamin D deficient (Brumbaugh, et al., 1982; Doetsch, et al., 2004; Omeroglu, et al., 1997). Still unknown is whether taking a higher than recommended dose would result in better outcomes.

Electrical stimulation and electromagnetic fields are treatment modalities that have been shown to increase the rates of bone growth and fracture healing through the induction of an electrical current or an electromagnetic field. Most of the studies in the scientific literature report outcomes from acute traumatic fractures that have failed to unite (nonunion fractures). For example, in 1990 Sharrad published a study using electromagnetic fields on tibial fractures that were slow to heal. The trial took place over a 12-week period and had a successful union rate of 45% in the treatment group compared to only 14% in the placebo group. Similarly, Scott and King (1994) reported a 60% success rate in the healing of nonunion fractures over 21 weeks with the use of capacitive-coupled electrical fields as compared to no treatment success in a placebo group. Unfortunately, because the nature of stress fracture healing is very different from that of other (complete) fracture types, it is uncertain whether these treatments would have the same beneficial effects.

There is limited evidence to support the effectiveness of low-intensity pulsed ultrasound (LIPUS) for reducing the healing time of stress fractures. Ultrasound is a form of mechanical radiation that can be transmitted into the body as high-frequency acoustical pressure waves. LIPUS units are small and portable and can be used independently by a patient at home. The LIPUS device consists of three components: (1) a plastic retaining and alignment fixture which allows the transducer module to be stabilized over the fracture site, (2) a battery-operated treatment module that supplies the low-intensity pressure waves, and (3) the control element, which is 110/220 V AC powered. A coupling gel must be applied over the treatment field. Treatment parameters are determined by a health care provider, but are typically daily 20 minute sessions composed of a burst width of 200 µs containing 1.5 MHz sine waves and a repetition rate of 1 kHz. Ultrasound has been shown to have the potential to favorably influence both inflammation and osteogenic activity (Heckman, et al., 1994; Brand, et al., 1999; Rubin, et al., 2001; Li, et al., 2007). Again, however, there is limited evidence to support its usefulness in the healing of stress fractures.

Summary

To successfully manage patients with stress fractures it is crucial to identify the reason the injury occurred in the first place. Intrinsic and extrinsic factors are often synergistic but nutritional factors including energy deficit, low calcium intake, and low-fat diets are common. As a consequence of energy imbalance and poor nutrition, reproductive hormone levels as well as growth factors known to support bone decline. Poor running technique and inadequate muscular support for the skeleton appear to be the most frequent catalysts of stress fractures.

Prognosis for the resolution of a stress fracture is excellent, provided the nutritional, hormonal, and mechanical factors can be addressed. The actual amount of time required for a fracture to heal depends on both location and severity. During the acute phase of the injury, the primary method of treatment is to reduce activity levels to the point at which pain is eliminated. The use of casts or non-weight bearing gait patterns should be avoided unless absolutely necessary to control pain and normalize gait.

It is important for athletes who feel they may be developing a bone injury to seek care immediately, as early intervention is associated with a quicker return to sport. Additionally, there are certain stress fractures that are prone to developing complications, including nonunions, for which more invasive care (surgery) may be necessary. Such fractures include but are not limited to the neck of the femur, the pars interarticularis (spine), the patella, the talus, the navicular, and the fifth metatarsal.

Comprehensive rehabilitation of the endurance athlete following stress fracture requires the resolution of all predisposing factors and the development or restoration of proper running technique. Special attention needs to be provided to the recovery of normal joint mobility, muscle flexibility, muscular strength/power, elasticity, and fatigue resistance.

REFERENCES

Adolphson P, Abbaszadegan H, Jonsson U (1993) No effects of piroxicam on osteopenia and recovery after Colles' fracture: a randomized, double bline, placebo-controlled prospective trial. *Archives of Orthopedic and Trauma Surgery* 112:127–130.

Albert M (1995) *Eccentric Muscle Training in Sports and Orthopaedics*. London: Churchill Livingstone.

Allen H, Wase A, Bear W (1980) Indomethacin and aspirin: effect of nonsteroidal anti-inflammatory agents on the rate of fracture repair in the rat. *Acta Orthopaedica Scandinavica* 51:595–600.

Altman R, Latta L, Keer R (1995) Effect of nonsteroidal anti-inflammatory drugs on fracture healing: a laboratory study in rats. *Journal of Orthopedic Trauma* 9:392–400.

Blick S, Dhillon S, Keam S (2008) Teriparatide: a review of its use in osteoporosis. *Drugs* 68(18):2709–2737.

Brand J, Brindle T, Nyland J, Caborn D, Johnson D (1999) Does pulsed low intensity ultrasound allow early return to normal activities when treating stress fractures? *Iowa Orthopedics Journal* 19:26–30.

Brumbaugh P, Speer D, Pitt M (1982) 1-alpha, 25-Dihydroxyvitamin D3 a metabolite of vitamin D that promotes bone repair. *American Journal of Pathology* 106:171–179.

Doetsch A, Faber J, Lynnerup N, Watjen I, Bliddal H, Danneskiold-Samsoe B (2004) The effect of calcium and vitamin D3 supplementation on the healing of the proximal humerus fracture: a randomized placebo-controlled study. *Calcified Tissue International* 75(3):183–188.

Eyestone E, Fellingham G, George J, Fisher A (1993) Effect of water running and cycling on maximum oxygen consumption and 2-mile run performance. *American Journal of Sports Medicine* 21:41–44.

Heckman J, Ryaby J, McCabe J (1994) Acceleration of tibial fracture healing by non-invasive low-intensity pulsed ultrasound. *Journal of Bone and Joint Surgery, American Volume* 76:26–34.

Holzer G, Majeska R, Lundy M, Hartke J, Einhorn T (1999) Parathyroid hormone enhances fracture healing. A preliminary report. *Clinical Orthopedics and Related Research* 366:258–263.

Li J, Waugh L, Hui S, Burr D, Warden S (2007) Low-intensity pulsed ultrasound and nonsteroidal anti-inflammatory drugs have opposing effects during stress fracture repair. *Journal of Orthopedic Research* 25(12):1559–1567.

Milgrom C, Finestone A, Novack V (2004) The effect of prophylactic treatment with risedronate on stress fracture incidence among infantry recruits. *Bone* 35:418–424.

Omeroglu H, Ates Y, Akkus O (1997) Biomechanical analysis of the effects of single high-dose vitamin D3 on fracture healing in a healthy rabbit model. *Archives of Orthopedics and Trauma Surgery* 116:271–274.

Reuben S, Ablett D, Kaye R (2005) High dose anti-inflammatory drugs compromise spinal fusions. *Canadian Journal of Anesthesia* 52:506–512.

Reuben S, Ekman E (2005) The effect of cycoloxygenase-2 inhibition on analgesia and spinal fusion. *Journal of Bone and Joint Surgery* 87A:536–542.

Rubin C, Bolander M, Ryaby J, Hadjiargyrou M (2001) The use of low-intensity ultrasound to accelerate the healing of fractures. *Journal of Bone and Joint Surgery* 83:259–270.

Scott G, King J (1994) A prospective double blind trial of electrical capacitive coupling in the treatment of non-union of long bones. *Journal of Bone and Joint Surgery, American Volume* 76:820–826.

Sharrad W (1990) A double blind trial of pulsed electromagnetic fields for delayed union of tibial fractures. *Journal of Bone and Joint Surgery, British Volume* 72:347–355.

Stewart G, Brunnet M, Manning R (2005) Treatment of stress fractures in athletes with intravenous pamidronate. *Clinical Journal of Sports Medicine* 15:92–94.

Swenson E, DeHaven K, Sebastianelli W, Hanks G, Kalanek A, Lynch J (1997) The effect of a pneumatic leg brace on return to play in athletes with tibial stress fractures. *American Journal of Sports Medicine* 25:322–328.

Zwas S, Elkanovitch R, Frank G (1987) Interpretation and classification of bone scintigraphic findings in stress fractures. *The Journal of Nuclear Medicine* 28(4):4452–4457.

GLOSSARY

Absorptiometry: A technique used for measuring bone density by exposing a bone to radiation and determining the degree of absorption. This is the technique that is used in a DEXA scan.

Acidosis: The condition in which arterial blood pH level is below 7.4.

Actin: One of the filament proteins within a sarcomere, interacting with myosin to produce muscle contraction.

Acute: In reference to inflammatory responses, these are the responses which are temporary and functional.

Adaptation: The capacity of the body and mind to accommodate to various physical and physiologic stresses.

Adaptive immune system: The complex of specialized cells and mechanisms that prevent or eliminate challenges from pathogens.

Adenosine triphosphate (ATP): The body's terminal chemical source of energy for muscular contractions.

Aerobic (aerobic pathway): Exercise metabolism that utilizes oxygen, involving the interaction of two interactive metabolic pathways: the Krebs cycle and the electron transport chain.

ALA: See alpha linolenic acid.

Alkalosis: The condition in which arterial blood pH level is above 7.4.

Alpha linolenic acid (ALA): Most abundant plant-derived form of omega-3 fatty acid.

Amenorrhea: The absence of menstruation in a female. This condition is most likely related to negative energy balance in a female athlete.

Amino acids: Chemically variant building blocks linked by peptide bonds to form proteins.

Anabolism: Metabolic activity that constructs larger molecules from smaller units.

Anaerobic: High intensity exercise metabolism that is possible in the absence of oxygen.

Anaerobic alactate pathway: Following exhaustion of regular ATP supply in muscle, derivation of additional ATP via chemical changes to creatine phosphate.

Anaerobic lactate (glycolytic) system: ATP formation via degradation of glucose or glycogen in the absence of oxygen.

Androgens: Male reproductive hormones such as testosterone.

Anemia: Lower than normal amount of red blood cells or hemoglobin in the blood.

Anorexia athletica: The condition in athletes who engage in unhealthy behaviors to control body weight (fasting, vomiting, excessive training).

Anorexia nervosa: A psychological disorder in which an individual restricts food intake in attempt to relentlessly pursue thinness. Compulsive endurance exercise often accompanies anorexia as a means to expend calories.

ATP: See Adenosine triphosphate.

Antioxidant: A molecule that is capable of preventing or slowing the oxidation of other molecules.

Antiresorptive drugs: Medications that reduce bone resorption by decreasing osteoclast activity.

Aromatization: Conversion of testosterone to estrogen in the bodies of males.

Atherosclerosis: The condition in which fatty material accumulated along arterial walls thickens and hardens due to calcification.

Basal metabolic rate: The amount of energy required to maintain physiologic processes of the body while at rest.

Bioavailability: The fraction of the total amount of an ingested nutrient or other substance that actually can be used metabolically by the body.

Biologic value (of protein): The proportion of absorbed protein from a food source that is utilized for maintenance and growth.

Bisphosphonates: A class of medications that reduce bone resorption. Alendronate (Fosomax) is a bisphoshonate.

BMR: See basal metabolic rate.

Body Mass Index (BMI): The ratio of body weight (kg) to height (m), which is often used to describe physical size in research settings.

Bone mass: Amount of bone mineral present in the body or in a particular location.

Bone Mineral Density (BMD): Amount of bone mineral in a given unit of bone area. Generally expressed as grams per centimeter squared (g/cm^2).

Bone remodeling: The process by which the skeleton repairs, maintains, and adapts. The typical remodeling cycle is characterized by the resorption of old or damaged bone by osteoclasts followed by the deposition of new bone by osteoblasts. A typical remodeling cycle requires several months to complete.

Branched chain amino acid (BCAA): Certain amino acids having branched side chains in their molecular structures, required for the metabolism of both carbohydrate and fat.

Cadence: Term used to describe the revolutions or cycles per minute of the various endurance sports.

Calcitonin: A hormone that inhibits bone resorption by acting on osteoclasts, available as a prescription medication (Miacalcin) for the treatment of osteoporosis.

Calcium: The major mineral constituent of bone tissue. Additionally, it plays a vital role in many body processes including muscle contraction. Calcium is often deficient in the diet of athletes. Dietary sources of calcium include dairy products and green leafy vegetables.

Calorie (c): The quantity of heat required to raise the temperature of 1 g of water by 1degree Celsius.

Calorimeter: A specially constructed chamber designed to measure the quantity of heat liberated by a body over a given period of time.

Capillary: Smallest division of the circulatory system in which nutrients and waste are exchanged between blood and tissues.

Carbohydrate loading: A dietary practice that involves ingestion of primarily carbohydrate fare in attempt to super saturate muscle glycogen levels in order to promote improved endurance performance.

Carbohydrates: Organic molecules including sugars and starches, composed of carbon, hydrogen, and oxygen.

Catabolism: Result of metabolic pathways that break larger molecules down into smaller units, releasing energy in the process.

Central nervous system (CNS): The part of the nervous system comprising the brain, spinal cord, and retina.

Chronic: A persistent or lasting condition or disease.

Circadian rhythm: A cycle of approximately 24 hours in behavioral, biochemical, and physiological processes of living organisms.

CK: See creatine kinase.

CNS: See central nervous system.

Coenzyme Q10: An oil soluble material present chiefly in mitochondria that is part of the electron transport chain in aerobic cellular respiration that generates energy in the form of ATP.

Computerized axial tomography (CAT): A test that can measure bone density as well as provide information about bone quality.

Cortical bone: The dense outer layer of bone.

Cortisol: A hormone produced by the adrenal glands in response to stress or exercise that can be detrimental to bone.

Creatine: A nitrogenous compound made from certain amino acids, important in muscle metabolism.

Creatine kinase (CK): An enzyme that uses ATP to break down creatine; levels are elevated in serious muscle breakdown as in myocardial infarction (heart attack) and other disorders.

CRP test: Medical assay for c-reactive protein, a general marker for infection and inflammation.

Cytokines: A category of signaling molecules, comprising small proteins secreted by the immune system and glial cells.

Daidzein: A type of isoflavone inherent in soy that is thought to be beneficial to bone health.

Deoxypyridinoline: Cross-linked form of type I collagen that is excreted in the urine and hence is a specific marker of bone resorption.

DEXA (or DXA): Dual energy X-ray absorptiometry, the most common test for measuring bone mineral density.

DHA: See docosahexaenoic acid.

Docosahexaenoic acid (DHA): Longer-chain form of omega-3 fatty acid.

Dual energy X-ray absorptiometry (DEXA): The most common test used to measure bone density. This test can measure total body bone mineral density as well as specific bones (hip, spine, forearm).

Eicosapentaenoic acid(EPA): A longer-chain form of omega-3 fatty acid.

Electrolytes: Substances that contain free ions producing electrical conductivity.

Elemental calcium: Actual amount of calcium contained in a food or supplement.

Endocrine gland: A gland that secretes hormones directly into the bloodstream rather than through a duct.

Energy balance: Functional steady state in which energy intake and energy expenditure are evenly matched.

EPA: See eicosapentaenoic acid.

Essential amino acids: Amino acids that cannot be synthesized by organisms (in this case, humans) and consequently must be present in the diet.

Estradiol: One of the forms of the hormone estrogen.

Estrogen: A reproductive hormone that is involved in many body processes including skeletal remodeling; considered to be a primarily female hormone but found in both genders, estrogen has different forms including estradiol, estrone, and estriol.

Fast twitch fiber (FT): A muscle fiber characterized by fast contraction time, low aerobic (endurance) capacity, high anaerobic capacity, ideally suited for high powered activities.

Fats: Organic compounds that are composed chemically of glycerol and fatty acids; serve as a concentrated source of calories.

Fatty acids: Chains 4 to 28 carbon atoms in length that end in a carboxylic acid group; major chemical component of fats.

Female athlete triad: A complex common in young women, comprising disordered eating resulting in energy deficit, amenorrhea, and osteoporosis.

FFA (free fatty acids): Resulting from the breakdown of fats, these relatively small molecules can be transported in the bloodstream without any carrier to anywhere in the body where there is a need for energy.

Flavonoids (isoflavones): The most common polyphenolic compounds in the human diet, believed to possess antioxidant activity.

Free radical: An atom or molecule that has a single unpaired electron in its outer shell.

Free Radical Theory of Aging: The concept that aging related to the accumulation of free radicals (outer shell unpaired electrons).

Genisten: A type of isoflavone inherent in soy that is thought to be beneficial to bone health.

Glucose: A simple sugar that represents the end stage product of carbohyrdrate metabolism.

Glycemic Index: A system of describing a food based upon how quickly it raises blood glucose levels.

Glycogen: The form in which carbohydrate is stored in the liver and muscle.

Gonadotropin releasing hormone (GnRH), also Leutinizing-hormone-releasing hormone: Is synthesized and released from neurons within the hypothalamus, and is responsible for release of follicle-stimulating hormone (FSH) and leutinizing hormone (LH) from the anterior pituitary.

Growth hormone: A hormone produced by the pituitary gland that stimulates bone and muscle development.

Homeostasis: Tendency of a system to regulate its internal environment and maintain a stable, constant state.

hs-CRP test: See High sensitivity CRP test.

Hydrogenated: Added pairs of hydrogen atoms to a molecule, in the process transforming double bonds between carbon atoms to single bonds; complete hydrogenation converts unsaturated fatty acids to saturated ones, in the process creating trans-isomers that have been implicated in circulatory diseases.

Hydrolysis: Splitting of a chemical compound into parts by addition of component elements of water (usually hydrogen and a hydroxyl group).

Hypercalcemia: Excess calcium in the blood, leading to a variety of symptoms including constipation, bone pain, fatigue, etc.

Hyperinsulinemia: Overly high levels of insulin in the blood; can cause hypoglycemia.

Hyperplasia: Increase in the numbers of muscle fibers.

Hypertrophy: Increase in size of individual muscle fibers.

Hypoglycemia: The metabolic state produced by a lower than normal level of blood glucose.

Hypogonadism: Decreased function of gonads, in which these glands produce little or no hormones.

Hypothalamus: Small, cone-shaped structure in the brain, projecting downward and ending in the pituitary gland.

Inflammatory response: Fundamental response to various injuries and diseases, symptoms including pain, heat, redness, and swelling.

Innate immune system: Evolutionarily ancient system of bodily defense involving cells (e.g. white blood cells) and molecules (e.g. cytokines) that defend the host against infection.

Insulin: Hormone central to regulating energy and glucose metabolism in the body.

Interleukin-1 (IL-1): Protein produced by various cells including macrohages, raising body temperature and spurring production of interferon and disease-fighting cells.

Interleukin-6 (IL-6): Secreted by T-cells and macrophages; acts as both a pro- and anti-inflammatory cytokine.

Interval training: A method of training that involves alternating higher intensity exercise segments with active rest or recovery periods. The high intensity segments are generally of relatively short duration but cumulatively allow for more total work than would otherwise be possible if the exercise was continuous.

Intramuscular lipid (intramuscular triglyceride, IMTG) stores: Lipids marbled among muscle fibers, serve as important supplementary store of energy during exercise.

Ironman: Worldwide competition in three events (swimming, biking, and running) held in Kailua Kona, Hawaii.

Isocaloric: Ingested food or beverages matched energy content, as for experimental trials.

Isoflavone: A compound, found mainly in soy foods and flax seeds, that produces estrogen like effects in the body.

Isometric: Resistance exercise in which effort expended by one set of muscles is opposed to that of another set.

Kaizen: Japanese philosophy underlying continuous improvement of processes.

Kilocalorie (C): 1,000 calories (c).

Kilojoule: 1,000 Joules, with one Joule representing the force of one Newton through a distance of one meter.

Lactate: An intermediate link between aerobic and anaerobic metabolism that is used as a marker of exercise intensity. The amount of lactate present in blood is correlated with reductions in pH levels (acidosis).

Lactate threshold: The intensity level in which during graded exercise lactate production starts to exceed lactate clearance.

LDL: See low-density lipoprotein.

Lactate dehydrogenase (LDH): Enzyme that catalyzes the interconversion of pyruvate and lactate.

Lactic acidosis: Buildup of lactic acid in the bloodstream faster than its removal, characterized by low pH in body tissues.

Ligand: A substance that binds to another molecule and serves as a trigger signaling mechanism.

lipolytic training: Strenuous endurance training resulting in reduced lipid levels.

Long slow distance training (LSD): A form of endurance training that is characterized by relatively low intensity sustained efforts.

Low-density lipoprotein (LDL): One category of size-graded lipoproteins, high LDL levels are believed to indicate susceptibility to atherosclerosis.

Low intensity pulsed ultrasound (LIPUS): Process that stimulates bone growth and aids healing of fractures.

Luteinizing hormone (LH): Hormone produced by the anterior pituitary; surge in this can trigger ovulation in females and Leydig cell production of testosterone in males.

Magnesium: A dietary mineral involved in ATP production, inflammation, and bone health. DRI is 320–420 mg/day.

Melanin: Pigment derived metabolically from the amino acid tyrosine; occurs in a variety of forms and concentrations, influencing skin color.

Menarche: The onset of menstruation.

Menopause: The cessation of menstruation.

Metabolic acidosis: Results from the body producing too much acid or the kidneys not removing enough; due to diverse causes and having consequences some of which are serious.

Metabolism: The set of chemical reactions in living organisms serving to maintain life; organized into metabolic pathways in which enzymes catalyze the stepwise conversion of precursors into products.

Milk-alkali syndrome: A condition caused by the ingestion of large quantities of calcium and absorbable alkali resulting in hypocalcemia.

Mitochondria: Tiny, membrane-enclosed organelles within which is generated most of a cell's supply of ATP.

Monounsaturated fat: Molecule composed of glycerol plus fatty acid with one double bond along chain of carbon atoms.

Monounsaturated fatty acid (MUFA): Fatty acid with one double bond along chain of carbon atoms.

Morton's toe: A common variant of human foot form in which the first metatarsal is shorter than the second metatarsal.

Motor unit: The set of a specific muscle fiber and the afferent nerve that innervates it.

MPO: See myeloperoxidase

MUFA: See monounsaturated fatty acid.

Muscle cross-sectional area (CSA): The extent of a theoretical slice of a muscle taken at the maximum thickness perpendicular to its long axis, serving as an indication of its propeties in contraction.

Myeloperoxidase (MPO): An enzyme, the breakdown products of which kill bacteria.

Myofibrillar hypertrophy:
Increase in size of muscle
subunits through increase
in the volume of contractile
proteins.

Myosin: One of the filament
proteins within a sarcomere,
interacting with actin to
produce muscle contraction.

N-telopeptide of type I collagen:
Specific breakdown product
of type I collagen found in
cartilage, and hence serves as a
marker of bone turnover.

**Nonsteroidal anti-inflammatory
drugs (NSAID):** Category
of drugs that reduce pain,
fever, and inflammation; most
are inhibitors of the enzyme
cyclooxygenase (COX),
so also are referred to as
COX-inhibitors.

One repetition max (1RM): The
maximum amount of weight
that can be lifted in a single,
successful exercise movement.

OPG : See osteoprotegrin.

Osteoblast: Specialized bone cells
responsible for bone formation.

Osteoclast: Specialized bone cells
responsible for bone resorption.

Osteopenia: A state of bone mass
that is below normal. Defined
statistically by bone mass that
is between 1 and 2.5 standard
deviations below the mean for
healthy young adults.

Osteoporosis: A state of bone mass
that is well below normal.
Defined statistically by bone
mass that is greater than 2.5
standard deviations below the
mean for normal young adults.

Osteoprotegerin (OPG): A
molecule that is involved in
bone cell remodeling, serving
as an osteoclast inhibitor.

Overload: A training stimulus that
exceeds an athlete's current
level of fitness.

Overreaching: The state in which
athletes are failing to adapt
to training demands. If the
circumstances are prolonged
it may result in the athlete
becoming overtrained.

Overtraining: A deep state of
fatigue that manifests itself in
both emotional and physical
ways that is presumably
related to endurance training
or racing in a manner that
exceeds an athlete's capacity to
adapt.

Oxalate/oxalic acid: Compounds
commonly found in plants
including buckwheat, rhubarb,
black pepper, parsley, etc.

Oxidation: A chemical reaction
that transfers electrons from a
substance to an oxidizing agent.
Oxidation reactions produce
free radicals that damage cells.

Oxidative stress: Imbalance
between production of reactive
oxygen molecules and ability of
the body to repair the resulting
damage.

Pamidronate: A nitrogen-
containing phosphanate said to
prevent osteoporosis.

Parathyroid hormone (PTH):
A hormone released by the
parathyroid glands in response
to low blood levels of calcium.

Peak bone mass: The greatest
amount of bone that an
individual acquires, a state that
generally is assumed to occur
during early adulthood.

Periodization: The process of compartmentalizing a training program into discrete but interrelated segments that emphasize certain aspects of an athlete's development.

pH: Literally "potential of Hydrogen" that serves as a measure of the relative neutrality, acidity, or alkalinity of substances, including the blood.

Phosphocreatine: Serves as a rapidly mobilizable reserve of high energy phosphate in muscle and brain.

Phytoestrogens: Compounds found in soy that produce effects similar to the hormone estrogen.

P1NP: A marker of bone formation, the full name of which is type 1 procollagen with an NH_2 terminal unit.

Pituitary gland: The gland that produces various hormones including follicle stimulating hormone and thyroid stimulating hormone that have important effects on the reproductive axis and bone.

Placebo: A simulated medical procedure that mimics the appearance of a treatment that is being tested.

Pleiotropic: Pleio (many) + tropism (an innate response); multiple effects of a single gene.

Plyometrics: A type of exercise training designed to produce fast, powerful muscle movements by loading and contracting a muscle in rapid sequence.

Polysaccharide: Organic molecule comprising a chain of multiple sugar subunits.

Polyunsaturated fat: Molecule composed of glycerol plus fatty acid with more than one double bond along chain of carbon atoms.

Polyunsaturated fatty acid (PUFA): Fatty acid with more than one double bond along chain of carbon atoms.

Pose running technique: A system for teaching human movement based on the ability of particular key positions to integrate a chain of action into an integrated whole.

Potassium: Dietary mineral that is important in pH regulation, exercise metabolism, and bone health. DRI is 4,000 mg per day.

Potential renal acid load (PRAL): Calculated values of certain foods that have the capacity to change the acidity or alkalinity of the body.

Power: In biomechanics, the product of force and speed.

Progesterone: A hormone produced by the ovaries.

Prohormone: Precursor substance to a hormone that usually has minimal hormone action itself.

Pronation: Inward rotation of the foot during normal motion.

Prostaglandins: Compounds that are synthesized in the body from fatty acid precursors which influence many body processes including the remodeling of bone.

Proteins: Nitrogen-containing organic food compounds

composed of amino acid units linked by peptide bonds.

PTH: See parathyroid hormone.

PUFA: See polyunsaturated fatty acid.

Quantitative Computer Tomography (QCT): Scans that produce virtual cross-sectional slices for observation of bone structures.

RANK: A molecular receptor located on the osteobloast, servng as an activator of nuclear factor KB.

RANK-L: A molecule that is involved in bone cell remodeling; specifically a ligand that is involved in osteoclast differentiation.

Rate coding: The frequency at which a motor unit is activated.

Rating of perceived exertion (RPE): A method of describing exercise intensity based upon an athlete's level of effort.

Recovery: A time dedicated to relative rest.

Repetition: The number of times a task is repeated. This may refer to the number of times a weight is lifted or describe the number of exercise intervals performed during a training session.

Repetition maximum (RM): The maximum load that an athlete can lift for a specified number of repetitions. A four (4) repetition maximum load is the amount of weight that can be lifted exactly four times.

Resorption: The phase of bone remodeling that involves bone breakdown.

Resting energy expenditure: The amount of calories needed by the body during a non-active 24-hour period.

Sarcomeres: Functional subunits of muscle cells, containing the filament proteins actin and myosin that are responsible for muscle contraction and relaxation.

Sarcoplasmic hypertrophy: An increase in muscle fiber size in the absence of an increase in the contractile proteins actin and myosin.

Saturated fat: A fat in which the carbon atoms in the molecule's backbone are linked by single bones, related to a high degree of hydrogenation.

Scoliosis: A medical condition in which the spine of a person is curved from side to side.

Set: A group of repetitions of a given exercise.

Sex hormone binding globulin (SHBG): A glycoprotein that binds to testosterone and estradiol during transport in the bloodstream.

Size principle of muscle recruitment: Small motor units are recruited first during low intensity exercise or for low force requirements.

Slow twitch fiber (ST): A description of a muscle fiber or cell that is characterized by slow contraction time, low force development, and high fatigue resistance.

Stress fractures: Incomplete breaks in bones commonly caused by repetitive stress.

Substance P: Neuropeptide related to the perception of pain.

Sugars: Sweet tasting, water soluble crystalline carbohydrates, most commonly monosaccharides (fructose, glucose) or disaccharides (sucrose, lactose).

Super-compensation: Attainment of a newly heightened level of fitness following workout stress.

Supination: Outward rolling of the foot during normal motion.

T-Score: A statistical measure defining an individual's bone density as compared to a population of normal young adults.

Teriparatide: A synthetic form of PTH.

Testosterone: The primary male reproductive hormone. Considered important for muscle and bone development.

Thermic effect of food: Increase in energy expenditure due to the metabolic cost of processing food for storage and use.

Thyroid: A gland located in the neck that produces the thyroid hormones. These hormones control metabolic rate and bone remodeling.

Total antioxidant capacity (TAC): This value refers to the full range of antioxidant activity against various reactive oxygen/nitrogen radicals.

Trabecular bone: Type of bone tissue that is located beneath the outer layer of cortical bone. Trabecular bone also is known as spongy bone and is the location of the greatest percentage of bone remodeling activity.

Trans-fat: Unsaturated fats containing trans-isomers resulting from partial hydrogenation.

Triathalon: A multiple-sport endurance event combining swimming, cycling, and running over various distances.

Tumor necrosis factor alpha (TNF-α): Most commonly mentioned of the general category of tumor necrosis factors, it is a cytokine involved in systemic inflammation.

Ultrasound: A test that utilizes high frequency sound waves to determine bone density.

Unsaturated fat: A fat with a high proportion of double bonds between carbon atoms in the molecule rather than single bonds due to hydrogenation.

Ventilatory threshold: The point during a graded exercise effort in which breathing becomes labored or deepens.

Vitamin D2: Ergocalciferol.

Vitamin D3: Cholecalciferol.

VO$_2$ max: The capacity for oxygen use by the body during maximal exertion. Usually expressed as liters of oxygen consumed per kilogram of body weight per minute (ml/kg/min).

Volume: A description of training quantity per unit of time. The combination of exercise duration and frequency that may be expressed in kilometers, miles, or hours.

Ward's Triangle: An anatomic region of the femur (thigh bone) that is commonly evaluated during DEXA testing to report bone density.

Z-score: A statistical test defining an individual's bone density as compared to a population of normal adults of similar age.

INDEX

ABOUT THE AUTHORS

Tom Whipple has been working with both recreational and competitive athletes as an orthopaedic physical therapist for over 20 years. He holds academic degrees in Physical Therapy (Northwestern University) and Orthopaedics (Georgia State University) as well as a certificate in Mechanical Diagnosis and Therapy from the McKenzie Institute, USA. He was recognized as an Orthopaedic Clinical Specialist by the American Physical Therapy Association (2000) and was certified by Nicholas Romanov, PhD, as a Pose Running Coach in 2004. His clinical practice at Penn State Sports Medicine is dedicated to the prevention and rehabilitation of musculoskeletal injuries in athletes with a special interest in stress fractures. He has held university teaching positions and has provided continuing education courses for practicing clinicians across the United States. In collaboration with scientists from The Pennsylvania State University he is pursuing research related to bone physiology in response to different exercise, nutritional, and hormonal states. He is married to Jody where together in central Pennsylvania they are raising their two children, Jacob and Abbey.

Bob Eckhardt is Professor of Developmental Genetics and Evolutionary Morphology in the Department of Kinesiology at the Pennsylvania State University, where he is head of the Laboratory for the Comparative Study of Morphology, Mechanics and Molecules. He has been conducting and publishing research for over 40 years, specializing in the development and evolution of the human musculoskeletal system. His research has been supported by the National Institutes of Health, the Australian Research Council, and several private foundations. He has published numerous scientific papers and books, most recently *Human Paleobiology* (Cambridge University Press, 2000). His laboratory was part of a research team that proved that the origin of bipedal locomotion occurred two million years earlier than previously realized (six million years ago rather than four million years ago). Dr. Eckhardt was an active recreational runner for several decades before shifting to vigorous daily walking for a more optimum balance between cardiovascular and biomechanical outcomes.